The Day I Forgot – But Will Always Remember

Living With Sudden Cardiac Arrest

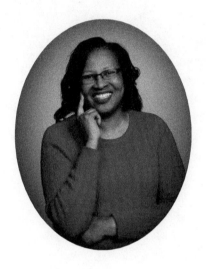

Dr. Brenda Brown
Flint, Michigan 48507

Scholarly Review

"Dr. Brown's account is incredibly moving and heartening, to say the least, to review one's own lifestyle and make changes and to have trust in a higher power. In reading her book, I found myself nodding my head at her story and the survivor stories truly realizing how lives can be changed instantly. She gives a wonderful opportunity to be a close-up witness on her journey from pain to restoration. Readers will be motivated and encourage to face life's challenge knowing someone like them made it through. A must read."

Mr. Twannie Gray, LMSW, CAADC, Solutions Behavioral Health (SBH), Saginaw, MI

~~~

"Dr. Brenda Brown's, "The Day I Forgot-But Will Always Remember...," Is a must read! This book provides awareness and critical information in such an intriguing manner. It is hard to put the book down once you begin reading. This book takes you on an incredible journey, as Dr. Brown very candidly shares her incredible challenges & triumphs with great transparency. We can all learn from her journey. Thank you, Dr. Brown for so generously sharing your story and the stories of others...This book has transformed how I view my own health and life."

Dr. Morris Thomas, PMP®, The University of the District of Columbia, Washington, DC

~~~

"Well articulated and heart felt acknowledgement of challenges and adversities we face in life. Dr. Brown is a strong, determined, caring young lady who has overcome many challenges in life relationship to her personal life, family situation, career aspirations and health as proclaimed in her book. This written testimony serves as motivation to others who are faced with similar challenges in their lives. Her desire to share her journey with "US" to enable others to achieve their goals and aspirations in life are of monumental importance to her and is articulated throughout the book. Her continued journey through FAITH and internal drive will serve as motivation to others. This is only the beginning, stay tuned for the next phase. Thanks for sharing your journey!"

Dr. LB McCune, Kettering University, Flint, MI

~~~

The Day I Forgot–But Will Always Remember
Brenda Brown, Ph.D.

ISBN 978-0-578-49342-8

Book Layout © 2017 BookDesignTemplates.com
Cover Design by Will Martin Designs
Cover Photo by JC Penny's Portraits-Lifetouch
Hair by Arlene Green, Salon In Season
Photos enhancement by Vision ENT Group/Anthony Naylor
Copyeditor: Darla Nagel

Scripture quotations noted KJV are taken from The New Scofield Study Bible. Authorized King James Version. Copyright © 1909, 1917, 1937, 1945, 1967 by Oxford University Press, Inc.

Survival stories in Chapter 4 are used with permission of the authors, Dave Olson, Lori Baughman-Lassen, Linda Hartleben-Wonder, Carol Mathewson, Tracy Clark, Nathaniel Brown, Britany Thomas, and Whitney Brown.

All photos published with permission.

Printed in the United States of America
By IngramSpark

The author is not responsible for websites (or their contents) that are not owned by the author.

DEDICATION

I dedicate this book to my children (Nathaniel, Britany, and Whitney), for letting me experience the kind of love that all parents wish for from their children, and to my mother (Marchel) and my sisters and brothers (Marcella, Linda, Mary, Dwight, Keith, James R., Lee, Eddie, Ricky, and Fred) for your endless and unwavering support.

ACKNOWLEDGMENTS

I acknowledge:
Ashley Knific, Rene McMann, Benita Seale, and John and Debra Collins for taking a knee by my side, to provide care for me that day. You each played an absolutely essential role in my outcome. You saved my life!

To Dr. K. Ahmed, Dr. E. Raj, and the doctors and nurses at Hurley Medical Center and U of M Hospital for not giving up on me! Your dedication and commitment saved my life!

My pastor (Rev. Jeffery Hawkins, Sr.) for your support and for walking the 10-mile route in tribute to me and the Prince of Peace Missionary Baptist Church family for your prayers and support. What an awesome God we serve!

The sudden cardiac arrest survivors who shared their stories with me for this book and the members of support groups, Sudden Cardiac Arrest and S.C.A. Survivor who support us all. Always remember to be strong and courageous. Do not be afraid or terrified because of what happened, "for the Lord thy God, he it is that doth go with thee; he will not fail thee, nor forsake thee" (Deuteronomy 31:6, KJV).

Contents

INTRODUCTION:

It Took a Brush With Death

❝An awareness of our own mortality can bring a sense of purpose to life. But all too often, that awareness comes in a way that is unexpected and terrifying" (Allan, 2013, para. 1). It took a brush with death to bring a sense of purpose to whatever time I have left. On one fateful day, August 14, 2016, I experienced a significant cardiac event that caused my own mortality to be at the forefront of my mind. The thought that I could cease to exist was and still is something I'm struggling with. The event is a reminder to me of just how fragile life is. This experience changed my outlook on life for better or worse.

A few months after my cardiac arrest, I had a counseling session with my pastor. I was struggling with my near-death experience and was having a difficult time adjusting to my rebirth. He told me, "Don't focus on what could have happened, but focus on what did happen!" He went on to say, "God spared your life for a reason...He has a purpose for you" (J. Hawkins, personal communication, November 2016). What

Pastor Hawkins told me then still resonates with me today. U.S. Representative Elijah Cummings, an American politician representing Maryland's 7th congressional district, said he would tell his children when questioned why something bad happened to them, "When bad things happen to you, do not ask the question 'Why did it happen to me?' Ask the question, "Why did it happen for me?" (*Baltimore Sun* staff, 2019, para. 5). As time goes on, I think often on these thought-provoking words and find myself growing more confident in my mortality and more able to maintain my mental and emotional stability.

Now, it still remains to be seen what long-term impact my brush with death may have. But for now, I have been transformed. My priorities are different. I have a fresh perspective on life: how I live, how I treat others, my appreciation of each day, and my renewed and strengthened faith in God. What I'm saying is that life has a way of knocking me down, but I got back up! You could say that this is kind of my own form of realistic optimism...to maintain a positive outlook within the constraints of life's hiccups...but it works. I'll get back up, and I'll continue to live my life...realizing that this is just one of many bumps in the road.

I live my life present to the moment I have been given. I no longer take for granted what was almost taken from me. My walk today is different from my walk before. I have a new normal. My book is, in essence, my process of defining what my new normal is.

My book describes my journey living as a survivor of sudden cardiac arrest (SCA). I wrote it more for my healing and to find my purpose. This book will forever be my reminder that my near-death experience was not the end of life but a new beginning.

I found a network of people, via the Sudden Cardiac Arrest Support Groups, who, like me, struggle with posttraumatic stress, cognitive challenges, and difficulty adjusting to our new reality. These struggles affect our temperament and influence how we interact with and respond to others. So, this book is also for SCA survivors as a reminder that when you are feeling overwhelmed with the difficult aspects of your encounter with death and of reentering this life, or you are in such a state where you don't know up from down and you can't spell your own name, you are not alone. Hopefully, this book will provide some answers. Finally, it is my hope that this book provides SCA survivors' family and friends with a better understanding and mindfulness of the challenges we deal with daily. When you tell us we should "just get over it," we need you to be kind and forgiving.

Chapter 1:
The Before - My Normal

M y "normal" was defined as being a mother of three, a grandmother to three, and a person who loved her family, friends and job. I woke up each day, went to work, faithfully attended church services on Wednesdays and Sundays, visited my family and friends, and never gave any thought about something bad happening to me. I never put a lot of thought into "Is tomorrow promised to me?"

I was born on September 27, 1957, at 5:12 p.m. to parents Jim and Marchel Brown. My parents did not know they were having twins until after my identical twin, Linda, was born and another baby (me) was pushing herself out. I am one of 13 siblings; two have passed away. I was born in Flint and moved to Otisville as a child. There, my siblings and I attended LakeVille Community Schools. After graduating from high school, I embarked on an encompassing professional and academic career that brought me back to the Flint area. After earning degrees from Hillsdale College, Central Michigan University, Baker

College, and Capella University, I immersed myself in Flint's postgraduate scene as the coordinator of the Academic Resource Center at Baker College of Flint. This was my normal.

Becoming an athlete started at my high school, where I ran track and cross country. I continued to run track and cross country during my college years at Mott Community College and Hillsdale College. After graduation, I continued to train and run in road races. Athleticism ran in my family. I have eight brothers and three sisters, and collectively, we played basketball, played softball, or ran track or cross country in high school or college, bowling leagues, and skiing. Two of my younger brothers, Eddie and Ricky, were talented runners and ran track and cross country for Saginaw Valley State University (SVSU). In fact, they were the main driving forces behind SVSU claiming back-to-back National Association of Intercollegiate Athletics Indoor National Championships in the 1982 and 1983 seasons. They still hold SVSU records for the hurdles, middle-distance runs, and relays, both for indoor and outdoor. In fact, Eddie tried out for the 1984 Olympics in the 400-meter hurdles.

After graduation from high school, I enrolled at Mott Community College. You can imagine my anguish when told that Mott did not have a women's track team. There was a men's track team but no women's track team. I vividly recall approaching the men's track coach to see if he was interested in forming a women's track team. He told me he was not. However, he did tell me that if I could gather together a group of ladies to form a relay team, he would allow us to practice with the men's team. Because the women's track team was not sanctioned by the college, we were unable to attend track and field meets with other female competitors. Nor were we able to compete against men at collegiate track and field meets. Society was not as accommodating of females competing against men back in the 1970s like it is today. Today, females can compete against men at the secondary and postsecondary levels with no pushback from society or any questions asked. The good news was that the coach allowed us to travel with the men's team to collegiate track and field meets when the event had both men and women competing. I was able to continue competitive running at Mott Community College.

In 1978, I transferred to Hillsdale College. I was a driven and determined athlete who strived continuously to beat my times. During my last year at Hillsdale, I was struggling to show up for practices. It became harder and harder for me to muster up the energy that would allow me to perform at my maximum ability. During track meets, I was literally dragging myself across the finish line, with my tongue hanging out, gasping for air. Something was wrong with me; I just didn't know what at the time. So, I made the decision to quit the team. It was devastating to give up something I enjoyed doing so much. I missed the camaraderie of my teammates. One month after quitting the team, I found out what was wrong. I was 6 months pregnant. Yes, 6 months pregnant! This explained my body's inability to muster up energy. You are probably asking, "Brenda, how could you not know that you were 6 months pregnant? Didn't you miss your monthly menstrual cycles?" My response to you is that it was not uncommon for me to miss my menstrual cycles during training. After all, I was running 10 to 13 miles each day for 5 to 6 days per week. My body was experiencing its own trauma from the hard workouts. I was a skinny young lady back then. Because I had run during the first 6 months of my pregnancy, I was small and was able to hide my pregnancy. I was 2 months away from graduating with my bachelor's degree and had every intention of walking across the stage. If the college administrators had become aware of my pregnancy, I would have been expelled from college and sent home. Prior to the 1980s, society was not as accepting of girls becoming pregnant out of wedlock. It was important to me that I finish my program and graduate with my class. So, I kept my pregnancy hidden. Two days after graduation, I gave birth to my first child on May 20, 1980.

After graduation, I continued to run competitively for 10 additional years in road races throughout my hometown. By the time my second child was born in 1990, I was married and working full-time at Hurley Medical Center (HMC) in the Cardiovascular Study Unit (CVSU). I was also enrolled in Central Michigan University's (CMU) master's degree program. After working 4 years in the CVSU, I was transferred to another department at HMC to work. There were four positions in the Health

Information Management Department that an employee could work. They were manager, coder, transcriptionist, and clerk. To work as a transcriptionist, as a coder, or in management, you needed an earned degree or certification in medical transcription, health information technology (HIT), or health information management (HIM), respectively. I did not have a degree in any of these specialty areas. In 1990, I requested a leave of absence from CMU in order to enroll in the HIT program at Baker College of Flint. I graduated from Baker College in June 1992 and sat for my certification exam in October 1992. Having successfully passed my HIT certification examination, I was promoted from clerk to coder. Three years later, I graduated with my master's degree from CMU.

As you can see, the demands on my time made it impossible to train competitively as a true athlete for road races. Again, I had to stop. I made a promise to myself that one day I would return to competitive racing. In April of 1992, I was offered a part-time teaching position at Baker College of Owosso. My third child was born in 1996. My life was drastically turned upside down when my husband and I divorced. All of a sudden,

I was thrust into the role of single parent. The stresses, such as having no one to tag in, self-doubt, making decisions solo, anxiety about money, and sleepless nights were taking their toll on me physically, emotionally, and mentally. Something had to give...but what? I made the decision to retire from HMC. I continued to teach part-time for Baker College until 1999, at which time I was offered a full-time management position. I had also applied and was accepted to Capella University's doctoral program.

~~~

The first signs that something was wrong with me began to manifest in late 2004. I was experiencing extreme fatigue coupled with vertigo, syncope, and dizziness. I was alternating between racing heart and shortness of breath. My anxiety level was off the chart. The fear of failure at this point in my career as a graduate student was causing me to feel overwhelmingly apprehensive. Even though I had passed my preliminary oral examination (proposal), I still had to get through the dissertation stage. For me, passing my dissertation defense would signify closure in my career as a graduate student and a significant milestone. It had been a long, strenuous, difficult, and tiring process that took me 6 years to complete. All I could think of was the conversation my academic advisor had shared with me and a class full of newly admitted doctoral students at our orientation: "A doctoral degree requires commitment and sacrifice." "Make sure this is what you want to do." "The worst thing you can do is finish the program and drop out at your dissertation stage." "Potential employers who see ABD [All But Dissertation] behind your name will think you do not finish what you start." My frustration level was higher than usual. Typically, I would run to manage my stress. Running was considered my quiet time, problem-solving time, and stress reliever.

My doctor diagnosed me with anxiety attacks. He explained that these symptoms would be short lived. Once I completed the dissertation stage of my program, this stressor would no longer exist, and my symptoms would go away. I accepted the diagnosis of anxiety attacks because I was under a lot of stress and his diagnosis made sense.

I continued to experience anxiety symptoms up to the date I defended my dissertation in February 2005 and was a candidate for my PhD. I was elated. By this time, my children were 25, 15, and 9 years of age. During the past 9 to 12 years, they had been incredibly patient and tolerant of the intensity of this process (working two jobs, earning my master's and doctoral degrees) and the time constraints that resulted in many sacrifices and a definite lack of family time. I appreciated their understanding and support and promised to spend more quality time with them. The stress I was under appeared to have evaporated, and life seemingly returned to normal once "we" walked across the stage to receive my degree and regalia in May 2005. I say "we" because of the sacrifices my children had made too. This was as much their degree as mine. I was officially done!

Unfortunately, in June 2005, I began to experience my symptoms again. On one particular occasion, the shortness of breath was so severe that I went to the emergency department. I was admitted for unstable angina and hypoxemia. My primary care physician stopped in to see me the next day, and I remember telling him that "something is wrong" and I was not leaving the hospital until he figured out what it was.

As an inpatient, I had numerous EKGs, an echocardiogram, and a chest X-ray. Nothing showed up. Having worked at HMC and having taught Quality Assurance in Healthcare at Baker College, I knew that hospitals were penalized by insurance companies when they kept nonacute patients in acute inpatient beds. I also knew that doctors could be penalized by the hospital and denied admitting privileges if they did not discharge patients when their status changed from acute to nonacute. I was no longer considered an acute care patient and was discharged from the hospital after 2 days. My primary care physician was no closer to finding out what was wrong with me. The symptoms I was exhibiting at home did not manifest themselves during my hospital stay. I did not want to leave the hospital.

I think more to appease me, my doctor scheduled an outpatient transesophageal echocardiogram for me the next day at Hurley's CVSU. The transesophageal echocardiogram is "a type of echocardiogram that uses a long, thin tube (endoscope) to guide the ultrasound transducer down the esophagus" (Emerson Hospital, n.d., para. 6) and that allows a closer look at the heart.

It was this test that shed light on why I was experiencing palpitations, shortness of breath, dizziness, and near syncope.

I was diagnosed with mitral valve prolapse (MVP). In layman's terms, everyone has two chambers on the left side of the heart: the left atrium and the left ventricle. "Your mitral valve, which is located between the two, is designed to allow blood flow from the left atrium into the left ventricle, but not back the other way" (Holm, 2018, para. 1). In my case, the flaps (cusps) of my mitral valve were not closing properly (thus, prolapsing) and caused a backflow into the left atrium during contractions (heartbeats).

My condition did not affect my daily lifestyle, nor was it serious enough to warrant surgery. I made some minor changes to how I moved through life, such as picking up heavy items to having someone else do it for me, running upstairs to walking upstairs, bending over from my waist to bending at my knees, and making sudden movements and/or jumping up quickly from a sitting position to moving more slowly. I was referred to a cardiologist, who told me that aerobic exercise (in moderation) would strengthen my heart and make it more efficient.

He recommended that I walk at a moderate pace for 30 minutes at a time. As a result, I continued my workout regimen and avoided lifting weights.

I functioned and led what I thought was a normal life with my MVP. I continued to work full-time for Baker College, taught Sunday school, and attended church worship services. I represented Baker College on a few community boards within Flint and Genesee County and spent quality time with my family. Life was working with me instead of against me. I was feeling stronger and energetic. With this new energy, I joined a cardio kickboxing class that met 2 days a week to help with strengthening my heart. Unbeknownst to me or my cardiologist, I was harboring a serious disease but was not experiencing any of the noticeable symptoms with which it is usually associated.

The disease finally manifested itself one particular day. It was a typical workday. It was a remarkable day. I did not experience any symptoms of fatigue, shortness of breath, near syncope, or chest pain. It was a good day! I left work at 5 p.m. and had dinner with my daughter before taking her to her karate class at 6 p.m. I sat and relaxed in the lobby area at her school while reading my book. When my daughter's class finished at 7:30 p.m., I changed into my workout clothes and began the process of stretching for my cardio kickboxing class scheduled to start at 8 p.m. Twenty minutes into my class, I started feeling extremely tired and was not functioning to my full capacity. My competitive nature would not allow me to appear weak in front of my classmates, so I left the room and went to the restroom to "gather" myself with every intention of returning to my cardio kickboxing class. It was there that my daughter-in-law found me kneeling over the toilet coughing up sputum. She said I was coughing up blood. I didn't see blood.

I refused her plea to call the paramedics and flat-out refused to go to the hospital by private car. "I'm okay," I told her. The instructor eventually came back and insisted that the paramedics be called too. I still refused. Besides, I told him, "What would it look like to potential students if they drove by and saw an ambulance in front of your school?"

After 10 to 15 minutes of persistent and constant persuasion, I opted to go to the emergency room by private car. I am insured with good health insurance from my employer. My focus was not on my health because nothing was wrong. My focus was on the emergency room bill I would receive in a few months for what I perceived as a nonemergency visit. Besides, I was feeling better and didn't need to be there. The triage nurse took my vitals and asked me how I was feeling. "Good!" I replied. I remember telling her that my daughter-in-law had insisted on me coming. The nurse wrote some notes on a sheet of paper, placed the paper in a canister, placed the canister in this automated transporter, and pressed the button that sent the canister to the back emergency treatment area. I was prepared to go to the waiting room to listen for my name to be called. Instead, I was immediately transported to a treatment room. The ER doctor came in right away. It was then that I knew something was wrong with me. I was in acute congestive heart failure, my blood pressure was dangerously high, and I had pneumonia. I totally lacked the signs and symptoms that correlate with the severity of the disease. I was admitted to the hospital from the emergency room. My journey in determining the extent of my heart disease had just begun.

~~~

"What were you doing?" my cardiologist asked. I replied, *"I was in my cardio kickboxing class. My daughter-in-law insisted that I come to the ER because she thought I was coughing up blood."* Needlessly to say, he was surprised because I had not consulted with him beforehand for clearance to enroll in the cardio kickboxing class. I knew my limitations with my MVP and was in tune, or thought I was in tune, with my body. My instructor was aware of my MVP and prohibited me from performing some of the routines. Even so, the class was too extreme for my heart.

During my inpatient stay, I had numerous EKGs, an echocardiogram, chest X-rays, and a cardiac catheterization done. I was given diuretics and spironolactone to treat my congestive heart failure and high blood pressure. I did not have coronary artery disease, my blood pressure was within normal range then, I was not diabetic, and I had no edema. I had not experienced shortness of breath. I was considered overweight but not obese. I reflected on the fact that there were absolutely no clues whatsoever that I was in heart failure. Mentally, this was overwhelming to me. I had a disease that shows no symptoms. What I did not know then but know now is that being asymptomatic would literally be the death of me when *it happened!* After my discharge from the hospital, I quit my cardio kickboxing class and made some additional lifestyle changes. I felt like a walking pharmacy as my cardiologist had me on beta-blockers, diuretics, and nitrates. I aggressively watched my diet to lose weight.

Family and friends would often tell me, "You have a really big heart," which is a delightful compliment except when it comes from my cardiologist. Having an enlarged heart often doesn't bode well, medically speaking. Unfortunately, my heart condition worsened, and I was diagnosed with hypertrophic cardiomyopathy (HCM). I found out that HCM's cause is genetic, more specifically, a genetic mutation affecting one of perhaps 12 genes. Each of the genes influences muscle formation, so in HCM, the heart muscle thickens, becomes disorganized, and develops fibrosis (forms scar tissue). "This thickening, along with other changes in muscle composition and function, can sap the heart's pumping power and can cause problems with its electrical system" ("Hypertrophic Cardiomyopathy," 2011, para. 4).

My cardiologist felt that heart surgery was inevitable in order to treat my disease. Surgical options were a septal myectomy or alcohol septal ablation. Both procedures, I was told, were effective in relieving symptoms and improving quality of life.

I opted for the alcohol septal ablation surgery because it was a less invasive surgical option than the myectomy. With the alcohol septal ablation procedure, a few drops of an alcohol-based solution is injected into the main artery to reach the thickened heart muscle using a small incision at the top of the leg. "This causes part of the muscle to die (in effect, a small heart attack) and this in turn reduces the obstruction to blood flow" (Stanford Health Care, n.d., para. 3). On the other hand, in a septal myectomy, an open-heart procedure, a surgeon removes part of the thickened muscle between the ventricles.

My heart surgery procedure was done on December 27, 2012, at Henry Ford Hospital. It took roughly 6 months before I noticed a difference in my symptoms. Although the surgical procedure did not alleviate my HCM, it did reduce the thickened muscle so that my heart could pump blood better. My symptoms were alleviated as I no longer experienced shortness of breath, dizziness, or syncope. My energy level increased. My heart appeared to be functioning better than before, and I was back to feeling what I defined as my "new normal." My heart was functioning well. Or so we thought.

~~~

Returning to regular athletic activity was also part of my "new normal." I decided it was time to participate in competitive road races again. I registered with the Crim Foundation to train with a team. All true athletes know that you cannot run or walk a race without training for it. For those of you who do not know, the Crim Festival of Races is an annual road running event with several races and walking events that has been held in August in Flint, Michigan, since 1977. The race attracts thousands of people each year from around the world. The first time I ran the actual 10-mile Crim road race was in 1977. The last time I ran the 10-mile Crim was in 1980, when I ran it in under 60 minutes. Since 1980, I've participated in numerous road races, in addition to playing on a softball league and bowling league. Back then before life got in the way, I was a true athlete in every sense of the word. I took my workouts seriously.

~~~

My cardiologist stressed the importance of not overexerting myself and told me to walk only, to take rest breaks often, and absolutely no running. This was a different mind-set for me. Historically, I had been a competitive runner, not walker. I was to go immediately to the emergency room if I experienced severe chest pains, extreme shortness of breath while walking, or any palpitations or feeling of syncope. I was to drink lots of water and stay hydrated.

I joined a Crim training team and trained on Tuesday and Thursday evenings. On the other days, I followed a training schedule provided by my team leader. I, along with a couple of my colleagues, would meet at Baker College at 6 a.m. on Mondays and Wednesdays to work out together. We would walk the streets within that community. When my colleagues could not meet me, I would stay on campus and walk the perimeter. Baker's Campus Safety officers would graciously keep a lookout for me via their cameras. This provided me with a level of security and safety, knowing that if I began to stumble, they would notice and come to my rescue. I maintained this same routine from June to August. On rainy days, I worked out inside the campus fitness center.

One of Crim's training guidelines was that participants had to compete in a minimum of three road races before the actual Crim road race in August. By mid-July, I had completed the minimum requirements. I felt pretty good and knew I was ready for the Crim. Two weeks prior to the actual race, Crim offers a practice walk/run of their 10K and 5K races the Sunday beforehand in order for race participants to gauge their readiness and time by running/walking the complete course. It also gives participants a glimpse into whether they have to make adjustments to their timing pace for each mile. There are hundreds of participants in this practice race. I had been training for this event and felt I was in shape to complete the race, not to mention conquer the famed stretch of steep inclines on Bradley Avenue at the 5-mile mark. Every athlete who has ever run the Crim road race knows about the Bradley Hills. They are the toughest part of the course.

The morning of Sunday, August 14, 2016, began as a typical Sunday for me. Normally, I eat breakfast, get dressed, and leave for church at 9:30 a.m. to teach Sunday school at 10 a.m. According to my daughter, Whitney, I appeared to be a little anxious that morning but attributed it to prerace jitters. The road race I was participating in began at 7:30 a.m. It was my intention to cross the finish line no later than 9:15 a.m. The night before, I had done a number of things. I had called and arranged to meet at my brother's house after the race to take a quick shower, change from my running gear, and head to church. I had loaded my car with my teaching supplies and a change of clothes. I had sent a text to my pastor and the superintendent of Sunday school about the race, informing them that I would be there to teach my class at exactly 10 a.m. I had downloaded Pharrell Williams's song "Happy" to my phone playlist. This song is very upbeat and full of energy. I had intentions of playing it as I climbed and conquered the infamous Bradley Avenue hills. I said goodbye to my daughter and left the house for the Crim practice road race. It was later that Pastor told me he remembered the text well. Jokingly, I had typed at the end of my message that I would be at class by 10 a.m. "unless I hurt myself and end up at Hurley Medical Center."

I do not remember arriving at the race or parking my car. I do not remember meeting up with my group leader at the clock tower as arranged. I was a volunteer to be a guide for a visually impaired walker. According to my team leader, Debra Collins, we initially met at the clock tower, a few feet away from the start line. She had left briefly to go get the athlete who was to walk with me. When she returned, I was gone. According to Debra, in hindsight, she noticed I was acting strangely but also attributed it to prerace jitters.

The race started and I had walked 8.8 miles when I collapsed. I do not have any memory of this day or of the next 3 days that followed. I've been able to piece together the details from family and friends. What I remember about my death and returning to what we call "this life" is waking up at the U of M Hospital, wondering why there were so many people in what I thought was my bedroom at home. I remember asking the people there, "What are you all doing in my room?" "Where am I at?" and "What happened?"

~~~

I was exactly 1.2 miles from completing the entire 10 miles of the Crim Festival of Races practice road race when I collapsed. I was elated that I had conquered the infamous Bradley Avenue hill, a hill so steep that if you stopped while walking or running it, you were likely to fall back down the hill. My team leader's husband (John) had walked with me. I had met John when he had attended some of the team training days. I praise and thank God for having John with me that day! John said we had met up with each other on the trail around the 3-mile mark. He said we talked as we walked. He had decided to stay with me because he felt something was wrong because I was not my usual self. According to John, I had finished the hills with no trouble. The hard part was over. I had called my son, Nathaniel, to celebrate because the biggest obstacle was behind me. I was excited because I knew I still had enough energy to walk the rest of the distance. John walked on ahead of me at the 8-mile mark. I was on my phone, and he felt I was okay. I have no memories of John walking with me or of calling my son.

According to Benita Seale, a witness walking behind me, I had just finished talking on my cell phone. As a rule, I never talk on my phone during a road race. But I did that day! I was on Miller Road, going toward the School for the Deaf, when Benita noticed that I seemed to be staggering somewhat. All of a sudden, I collapsed to the ground, motionless. I had lost consciousness before I hit the ground and was unable to brace for impact, smashing my face against the pavement.

Benita said she called out to God for help all while attempting to perform CPR. She said she didn't know what she was doing but had to try. As I was digging for details about that day and for this book, I found out that another runner, Eric Wisniewski, and his running partner had also rushed up to me. According to Eric's wife, Majory, Eric remembers the horrific sound of me hitting the pavement. He had rolled me over and then gotten out of the way so that CPR could be administered. He also helped find my ID for the emergency responders.

People were beginning to form around me. Standing, watching, and waiting. Within minutes of my collapse, Ashley Knific had walked up to the crowd of people surrounding me as I lay unconscious on the pavement. Unaware that 911 had been called, Ashley called 911 again, telling the operator, "There is a lady on the ground unconscious."

"Does she have a pulse?" the operator asked.

"She has a faint pulse," Ashley replied.

"Do you know how to administer CPR?" the operator asked.

"I'm certified but have not had to perform it on a person. It has been years. I don't know if I can do it," Ashley replied. The operator asked Ashley to put the phone on speaker and said she would walk her through it. Amid frantic assistance from other racers, and 7 months pregnant, Ashley started chest compressions.

Another racer, Rene McMann, walked up to the crowd of people surrounding me 3 to 5 minutes later. She noticed that Ashley was performing chest compressions and that she was slowing down and off count. She quickly got down on her knees next to Ashley, waited for Ashley to raise her hands in between compressions, and then gently moved her hands away – not skipping a beat – and continued CPR on me. I repeatedly took deep breaths, exhaled, and then stopped breathing. Eric watched as they lost my pulse three times before the paramedics arrived. My right arm kept jerking as if I were having a seizure. I was refusing to give up. *As long as this lady is not willing to give up, I will continue to work at keeping her alive,* Rene thought. Rene said she kept wondering why it was taking the paramedics so long to arrive. In the midst of any emergency, the wait for help to arrive always appears to be longer. No one knew who I was other than John. Fortunately, I had my emergency card with me in my pouch. The paramedics arrived, loaded me into the ambulance, gave my heart one shock treatment, and continued CPR. With my emergency card, the paramedics were able to identify who I was, my medical history, the medicine I was taking, my primary care physician's name, and my cardiologist's name. I was transported to Hurley Medical Center (HMC) as Brenda Brown alive and not Jane Doe dead on arrival. Thank God!

Benita had hopped into the ambulance with me. She was the link to my family. God was smiling down on me that day. Something you should know about me is that I have never talked on my phone during a road race in my entire life except on this day. Benita picked up my phone and pressed "Recent Calls" to redial the person she saw me talking to on the phone at the 7-mile mark. She did not know it was my son. She didn't know me, and I didn't know her. All she knew was that someone had to be told about me. My son, thinking I had redialed by mistake, initially was not going to answer the call. He was just stepping into the shower but decided to answer the call and was told that I had collapsed. His world and my family's world changed on August 14, 2016.

Upon arrival at Hurley's emergency room, I was immediately taken to the trauma treatment area, where I received care from highly skilled ER physicians. One day, I will go back and meet them. HMC was and is my hospital of choice, and I was happy I was taken there. My experiences at Hurley have always been positive. I worked there for 12 years and go there for medical care. Depending on whom you talk to, Hurley is a city hospital for indigent (poor and needy) patients. However, shamefully, I want to give a plug for HMC, which houses the only Level I Trauma

Center and Level II Pediatric Trauma Center (the highest designations possible), in the region. It offers the only Level III Neonatal Intensive Care Unit and hosts one of just six specialized burn units in the state. Hurley Children's Hospital provides exceptional clinical care in the form of nationally recognized pediatric and neonatal programs. Central to those programs is Hurley Children's Hospital, the premier medical facility in the region and a Children's Miracle Network Hospital since 1990. When it is a matter of life or death and you are near Hurley Medical Center, it is the place to go!

Doctors and nurses were surrounding me. In case anyone reading this really wants to know, there was no door to the other side...I didn't have my whole life flash by...no bright lights...no out-of-body experience. In fact, I don't recall anything about my stay at HMC because the first thing I recall after my sudden cardiac arrest (SCA) is a vague memory of waking up in the intensive care unit (ICU) 4 days later, at U of M Hospital in Ann Arbor.

After the call from Benita, my son drove from Redford, Michigan, to HMC. My daughters, Whitney and Britany, were called. My brother

Fred was also called. Fred called my mother and other siblings. Whitney called my pastor. My twin sister and my brothers, who lived in Mississippi, North Carolina, and Atlanta, were called and arrived early the next day. A social worker gathered the family together in a room, which my son describes as the room where "you tell family members their loved one was not expected to survive or had passed away." I was still unconscious. My family had not seen me yet.

I was transported to the ICU and placed on the post–cardio arrest hypothermic protocol due to the severe trauma to my body. This protocol improves mortality and neurological outcomes in patients who have survived cardiac arrest, with the goal being to maintain hypothermia (target temperature of 33°C) for 24 hours. My family was not able to see me until the day of the transfer to ICU, August 15. Because it still appeared that I was not going to survive, all my family members were allowed to come to my room. I can only imagine the anxiety and uncertainty they were feeling. Friends from the race were there as well. My oldest daughter called my ex-husband, a retired nurse from HMC, to inform him of what had happened. He came out for support. He and she (an anesthetist's assistant) oversaw my care, talked to the doctors, and translated the medical jargon into layman's terms to my family.

~~~

When I collapsed, I hit the pavement head first and suffered a fractured orbital bone. John, who had walked with me up to the 8-mile mark, said he was up ahead near the 9-mile marker when he heard a loud sound, like a pumpkin being thrown to the ground and busting open. He said he turned, looked, and saw a crowd beginning to form. He walked back to see what was going on and saw that I had fallen. He immediately called his wife (Debra), my team leader, and told her what had happened and that she needed to come back to the location right away. Debra, having just walked across the finished line, flagged down a police officer to take her to me.

As a result of the fall, my left eye was completely engulfed and had disappeared from the swelling. I also had a traumatic facial soft tissue injury with an open laceration and a contusion on the left side of my face. I was unconscious before I hit the pavement. If conscious, I would have been able to control my fall as I was taught in my cardio kickboxing class.

I did not feel any pain. My cardiologist and his team were treating my SCA. However, my face was so badly swollen that it was difficult for my ophthalmologist to ascertain what was going on. The nearest ophthalmologist who specialized in optical trauma to treat my orbital fracture was in Ann Arbor, Michigan. My primary care physician arranged to have me airlifted to University of Michigan Hospital in Ann Arbor on August 17, 2018, for treatment of the orbital bone fracture. The cardiologists at U of M would assume care of my SCA in conjunction with my cardiologist in Flint.

I remained in U of M's ICU for about 2 weeks. I was taken off the hypothermic protocol on August 18, 2016, per my oldest daughter's request. I was awake. I slowly began my recovery. My nurses had me up walking and sitting in a chair. My family was with me around the clock. I had numerous EKGs, echocardiograms, X-rays, and blood draws done. I had attending physicians and physician assistants in to see me seemingly every 4 hours. All of my nurses were nice with excellent bedside manners. I had one particular ICU nurse who was exceptional at her job. She was caring to me and my family. In fact, she felt like family.

When I was transferred to U of M's transitional unit, she would stop by to check on me.

By the time I was transferred to the transitional unit at the end of August, my prognosis was serious but stable – my vital signs were within normal limits under the circumstances and I was conscious. I was walking the hallways with the aid of a portable walker. My facial swelling had decreased significantly. X-rays were ordered and showed that I had a hairline orbital fracture that did not require surgery. According to the specialist, the fracture would heal on its own. The laceration was cleansed daily. Over time, the laceration closed, and an antibiotic ointment was used to lightly rub over the scar. I have a visible scar below my left eyebrow. Due to the traumatic facial soft tissue injury, my left eyebrow hair no longer grows.

As my condition continued to stabilize, the cardiologist informed me that I needed an implantable cardioverter-defibrillator (ICD). An ICD is a device implanted inside the body that can help control life-threatening arrhythmias by analyzing the heart rhythm and determining whether a shock is required. If a shock is required, an electric current (shock) is delivered to the heart by the cardiac defibrillator, which interrupts the chaotic rhythm and allows the heart to return to normal. A representative from the company, Boston Scientific, came in to visit me in my hospital room. He showed images of the device that would be implanted, showed where the device would be implanted, and answered any questions I had. Showing my ignorance of defibrillator implants, I should have asked why the implant was being placed in my back about 3 inches directly below my left armpit instead of in my chest above my heart. I did not ask because I thought it was a standard implant location. Does it bother me to have it there? No, not in the least. It hasn't caused me any problems in its current location.

My ICD was implanted on September 5, 2016. I would be lying if I told you the implant surgery did not hurt. I remember waking up in the operating room to the surgeon pressing on the ICD device incision site. I was taken off the anesthesia too soon. By the time I arrived back to my room, I was in tears. A nurse gave me something for pain, and I went to sleep. Although the doctor was ready to discharge me the next day, I remained in the hospital for 2 additional days because the pain from the ICD device and the incision site was excruciating. I was discharged on September 7, 2016. I went to my mother's house to recuperate. I was afraid to sleep in a room alone for fear of another SCA happening. My brother, Lee, had twin beds in his room and agreed to my sleeping in his room. My children and siblings came to my mother's house to visit with me. My brothers and sister who lived out of state had already returned to their respective homes prior to my discharge from the hospital. My mother and brother took care of me until mid-October. Then I returned back to my home with my youngest daughter and her 1-month-old daughter (My fourth grandchild, Nicole, who was born on September 24, 2016). While writing this boot, my fifth grandchild, Nyla, was born on February 25, 2018.

While recuperating at my mother's, I contacted my team leader to see if she could find out the names of the ladies who had performed CPR on me. I wanted to reach out to these ladies personally to say thank you and to find out what happened. She was able to contact them via the Crim Foundation office, and we all met for the first time for dinner in late November. The Crim

Foundation offered me the opportunity to finish the race where I left off. So, 2 months after my dream of completing the Crim road race was delayed when I went into cardiac arrest, I was able to pick up where I had collapsed and finally crossed the finish line on Thursday, November 5, 2016. I was recognized by the local news station, WJRT ABC 12, as its person of the week.

Before my cardiac arrest, I didn't give much thought about if something was going to happen to me, life, or death. I was (still am) a parent and grandmother. I woke up each morning, went to work, and performed my job responsibilities. I was actively engaged within my community and a strong supporter and defender of social injustices. I was a *Big* Sister to this *Little* girl through the Big Brothers/Big Sisters of Greater Flint. I was also an actively engaged member in my church. I was a mentor to college students and much more. Truth be told, I expected then (and still do) to live until I am 100 years old.

As a Christian, I know that our times are in God's hands. I also recognize that for some, their journey on earth is much shorter. I also know that no one evades death, no matter how strong they are or how many years they live. But God saw fit that this was not my time. Without a doubt, he placed Benita Seale, Ashley Knific, Rene McMann, and John Collins in my path that day. My faith is in him! So, why was it wavering? Why was I having doubts?

I found myself, out of fear, avoiding doing those things that I used to do. I questioned why God spared my life. Was there a purpose for my continued existence? I experienced anxiety attacks. I was afraid to drive for fear of my defibrillator firing off and losing control of my car. I experienced sleepless nights for fear of dying in my sleep. I had nightmares. Was fear causing my faith to waver? Was it causing me to have doubts?

I was struggling with everyday challenges, such as fatigue, getting dressed, taking a shower, walking, negative thoughts, failure to immediately process what was being said to me, and memory loss. I was not able to concentrate on a particular activity or topic for longer than 5 minutes because my attention span had significantly decreased. It was like my brain was blank. I was simply stuck! I could not walk for the first few months without the aid of a walker because my equilibrium was still off. I was unable to recall family and friends' names without pausing to think about it first. I knew the information was there, tucked back in my mind. I just couldn't get to it. I found myself writing everything down just so I could remember it. I found myself asking people to repeat what they had just said. Unlike having dementia or Alzheimer's, where you don't know that you don't know, this time was very scary for me because I knew that I was struggling to remember or recall names, events, or things.

What if it happens again? I would ask myself each morning. *What if it happens and I die?* During this time, my fears were my reality. My doctors reassured me that if it did happen again, I had the assurance that my defibrillator would protect me. Was I being irrational? I would remind myself that if God spared my life once, he could do it again. But, I had to ask the questions "Why did God allow it to happen to me the first time? How do I know if he will not allow it to happen again?" I realized that I had to strengthen my faith, get rid of my doubts, and make the most of life. I started my journey to my new normal.

The first major thing I did was return to work in November 2016. To alleviate worrying my family or raising concerns at work, I would hide how I was feeling behind a bright smile. I pretended that everything was okay. But in reality, it was not. I was working again, going out with friends, and basically living life, but this was for appearances. I still struggled with my faith and had my doubts. In the midst of my storm, I was diagnosed with another incurable disease.

Exactly 1 year after my cardiac arrest, I had a cardiology genetic study done at U of M Hospital in Ann Arbor. The purpose of the test was to determine whether heart disease is hereditary in my immediate family, and it is not. Cancer and diabetes are prevalent in my father's family. His father, mother, and siblings all died of either cancer or complications of diabetes. On my mother's side of the family, her brothers died of cancer and her mother of organ failure as a result of old age. Her father died from complications due to a fall.

The results from my cardiology genetic study were positive for late-onset transthyretin amyloidosis. I am part of the approximately 3–4% of the African American population who has the transthyretin pathogenic V124I variant. This gene mutation causes a slowly progressive condition that interferes with normal function of the organs because too much amyloid, a kind of protein, collects in them (Cedars-Sinai, n.d.).

Prior to my cardiac arrest, my neurologist had diagnosed me with carpal tunnel syndrome, pressure on the medium nerve. I was receiving corticosteroid injections every 3 months. After my cardiac arrest, the pain was unbearable. Thinking that when I hit the pavement I had irritated the median nerve, I didn't allow myself to dwell on it too much. I took Aleve for pain management. I figured in time the pain would go away, but it did not.

In July 2018, I was officially diagnosed with peripheral neuropathy. Peripheral neuropathy means damage of the nerves that run to the limbs (peripheral nerves). I had decreased sensation in my toes and fingers, making it difficult to walk and function properly. My neurologist prescribed gabapentin for pain management.

By this time, I was feeling very overwhelmed. I was diagnosed with two more incurable diseases, one of which did not have a Food and Drug Administration–approved treatment plan. My world was falling apart!

I was ready for some good news.

CHAPTER 3:

The Now: Living With Sudden Cardiac Arrest

T here used to be days when I suppressed all thoughts of that eventful day and the days that followed after my cardiac arrest, especially after looking at the photos and videos that my brother, Keith, had taken. I still have days when I am afraid to go to sleep due to this overwhelming fear of dying in my sleep, only to wake up the next morning and not feel like getting out of bed because of the overwhelming fear that on that day I will have another cardiac arrest and not survive. Even with repeated reassurance from my cardiologist that I am protected with my defibrillator, I was still fearful to the point of panicky. I was suffering from posttraumatic stress, cognitive challenges, and difficulty adjusting to my new reality.

My primary care physician recognized my symptoms of depression and anxiety. He recommended that I speak to a therapist for help with developing coping skills and how to process my emotions and feelings. Initially, I was hesitant about seeking help from a therapist because of the negative stigma that surrounds counseling, the stigma that says one must be "crazy" if they are seeking counseling. This stigma was a major deterrent for me in seeking help. I did not want others to think I was "crazy." I waited 2 years before I sought professional help for my depression and anxiety. Recognizing that my view of myself was more important than what others thought, I scheduled an appointment with a therapist. I now tell anyone who will listen that I am seeing a therapist and that my counseling sessions are useful to me. This is all that matters. My message to others is that if you are experiencing challenges in your life, do not sabotage yourself, based on unfounded stigmas, from taking the steps necessary to move forward in your life.

I am meeting with my therapist twice a month to learn how to cope with my emotions and feelings after experiencing sudden cardiac arrest (SCA). My therapist has helped me to tackle my fears and depression directly so that I am now able to see things more clearly. At one of my sessions, my therapist had me complete this exercise that was very helpful. He gave me a sheet of paper with three columns. The first column was labeled "Anxious Fear." I had to write down my fears in column 1, indicate the likelihood of my fears happening again in column 2, and write what I should focus on or do in (in regards to my fears) in column 3. This exercise forced me to focus on the facts and what is actually happening now, instead of what might happen in the future. Unfortunately, my fear of having another cardiac arrest has prevented me from doing ordinary things, such as driving long distances by myself (because my defibrillator could fire off while driving, causing me to lose control of my car), flying in an airplane by myself, being alone for extended periods throughout the day or overnight, and maintaining financial security (because I was on medical leave from work during the time this book was written).

The hardest part for me now is accepting that things will *never* be like they were. I know I will not wake up one day and have everything back the way it was. I have days when I am down and depressed and ask myself, "Why me? Why is this happening to me?" but then I think about the alternative and how I almost didn't make it to see my family another day. This thought gives me a new perspective.

When my faith began to waver, my pastor would pray for and with me. During my meltdowns, he would have me read from the book of Job and tell me that "God is up to something or the devil wouldn't be fighting you this hard!" You're going to win this"; and "Stay close to the fire!" I find strength and encouragement in scriptures and songs. I appreciate the small joys that pass my way.

My family is everything: my rock, my best friends, and my backbone. From day one, they have put their arms around me, supported me, put up with my mood swings, driven me to my doctor's appointments, financially supported me when I needed help, and simply just been there when I needed them. My youngest daughter moved back in with me so that I would not be alone. My oldest daughter interpreted everything the doctors told me in layman's terms so that I understood. If it didn't sound right to her, she would question the treatment plan. My son, the chef, would cook me meals so that I didn't have to bother with cooking.

I embrace my second chance at life. The opportunity to more fully appreciate the people, things, and experiences many of us take for granted. The chance to live for today, knowing tomorrow may never come. A time for new experiences and memories. And, the excitement of exploring new directions, to do bigger and better things.

I focus on eating healthier meals and on using brain training memory and game apps that allow me to assess and train my memory and concentration, as well as increase my cognitive skills. There are a number of free apps I'm using, such as Lumosity, CogniFit Brain Test & Training, Mind Games Brain Training, Solitaire, and Word Connect, that are helping me learn new habits of successful engagement with life.

Other apps that are free downloads from Apple that I use to relax, or to provide inspiration and motivation in overcoming my fears and to persevere in my daily walk with Christ, are the Calm app and Daily Bible Quote app.

I am a member of both the Sudden Cardiac Arrest Support and S.C.A. Support Groups, located on Facebook, where members share their stories and challenges. An SCA event is quite different from other tragedies because few people understand what SCA is or how their loved one came to be a victim. This group of survivors understand and can relate to how each member feels and the challenges we face on a daily basis. We all know that still being here is a definite plus.

There are no cures for the diseases my body has. Instead of dwelling on what can't be, I dwell on what is. Earlier in my book, I said that I needed some good news. What was in front of me all along, I did not see. The good news is that I am a survivor! My new birth, my new life, are positive signs that things will indeed work out.

I'm often told that God had his angels watching over me, that I am a walking miracle. I know that God is with me, He loves me, and everything is going to work out for my good. I also recognize that the fear and doubt I was experiencing was nothing but a tool the devil was using against me to make my life miserable. Satan tried to destroy my life by turning my back on God. But, God told Satan, "No, not this one!"

In writing this book, I found my purpose. In part, it is to explain to anyone and everyone who will listen about the hidden heart conditions that often are deadly. These conditions exist, they can be diagnosed, and lives can be saved.

My story is not finished; it is just beginning!

Christmas Letter
By Dave Olson

I'm on the road a fair amount for my job. Occasionally I have an event where I invite Cheryl to join me. In July it was a conference in Leavenworth, a town about 3 hours away. Initially she declined, but then the day before, she decided to join me. And because she did, I'm still able to write our annual Christmas letter.

On the first night, Cheryl awoke to some horrible sounds as I sat up in bed and was struggling to breathe. Then I slumped over. She called the hotel operator and said, "Call 911, my husband's not breathing!" Initially, she went a little old-school CPR on me, and gave me a few mouth-to-mouth breaths. It was a nice little romantic getaway to Leavenworth, so I think that was sweet. But then, the harsh reality set in as she realized I had no pulse. So she dragged my deadweight, cheeseburger-infused physique off the bed and started chest compressions. Snap, crackle, and pop she went with "Staying Alive" going through her mind just like she learned in her CPR class. She had to stop and rest occasionally, which allowed her time to go to the LinkedIn app on her phone and update her profile under "Skills" to add CPR. A sheriff's deputy overheard the 911 call go out and drove over to see if he could help. He was the first to arrive, so he tag-teamed Cheryl and took over, while she critiqued his technique. Next, the first responders from the fire department arrived – two 18-year-old recent high school graduates and a 19-year-old guy. They took over CPR from the deputy, who wondered to himself if these guys had even started shaving yet. The next crew to arrive were the paramedics, and before we knew it, there was a party in Room 205 with everyone taking turns doing CPR on me.

As Cheryl watched them work, the sense of relief that help had arrived quickly faded when they attempted, and failed, to restart my heart, multiple times. Eventually, another deputy who had arrived on scene politely escorted Cheryl out of the room. Ruh-roh. While they sat in the lobby, waiting, one of the comments the deputy made was "If they don't get a pulse, they won't transport." Wait, what? You mean those hunky fire department guys might just give up and tell Cheryl to call the coroner? Back in the room, I thought for sure I heard the guy working the AED exclaim in a Scottish brogue, "I'm givin' her all she's got, Captain." Fortunately, two of the beefcakes from the fundraising calendar, Mr. April and Mr. November, finally got my heart restarted, which actually surprised them. Apparently they don't arrive on scene very often to find a dead guy lying on the floor and bring him back to life. I guess it happens more in the movies than in real life.

Over at the hospital 30 minutes away in Wenatchee, my heart kept going into V-fib, a pulseless rhythm, also known as the death arrhythmia. Every time it did, Cheryl would be politely escorted out of yet another room. Someone else would then jump up on the gurney and start CPR. Fortunately, my wallet was still back at the hotel, so no one ever knew my organ donor status on the back of my driver's license. I kind of felt like Resusci Annie, although they hadn't amputated my arms and legs yet. In the cath lab they ruled out a heart attack. What, no heart attack? Awesome, no dietary restrictions. "I'll have some Animal Fries with my order." They actually found my heart to be quite strong. It was just that pesky electrical issue, or arrhythmia, known as V-fib. Fast-forward 23 days in the hospital later, a 3-day coma, 7 days on a ventilator, an ICD placement, an ablation procedure to zap some areas in my heart, and a few smuggled-in Blizzards for dietary sustenance, I was good to go. I was a little woozy the first few months, but today, I feel great. Totally 100% back to normal. I've already been back on the trails with a 12-mile hike under my belt. No hypoxic brain injury damage, despite opinions to the contrary when I was out of my coma and finally off the ventilator. (Sorry, girls, that your dad was acting a little wacky. I didn't mean to scare the bejeebers out of you like that. #thisisyourbrainondrugs.) A lot of doctors and rehab nurses involved in my care are still puzzled as to how I can be so completely normal after all that I went through, but for me, "normal" is a relative term.

Robyn lives in downtown Seattle in a cute studio loft. She works at an IT company in marketing and sales support and does some occasional modeling in her spare time. Since her company headquarters are near us, she occasionally crashes in our guestroom, so she was spending the night when Cheryl made the call home at 4 a.m. to let the girls know what happened. Cheryl had handed her phone to the deputy to give Robyn some directions on where to go, so it was Robyn who was told those infamous words to stay put for now because "If they don't get a pulse, they won't transport" as Cheryl overheard the conversation. Kind of an "Other than that, how was the play Mrs. Lincoln?" comment.

Robyn then woke Emily up with the blunt news "Dad doesn't have a pulse." It's still unsubstantiated at this time, but rumor has it Emily said "WTF?" (Mom – that's text language for "Why the Face?"). Okay, so maybe Emily didn't actually let loose with the queen mother of dirty words but only thought something along those lines. But you get the idea though. Then, after rousing Bethany, the three of them packed their bags in record time for three girls. As they were about ready to head out the door, the deputy called back to say I was alive. Lo and behold, they had transported after all. Bethany, who doesn't stress about much, was happy that they would now have time to go through a Starbucks drive-thru on the drive over.

Adria and Alex are currently working to pay the bills while they pursue their dream jobs. For Alex, it's a youth pastor position someday. For Adria, it's in the literary world as an agent. She spent the summer in NYC at Columbia University in their postgraduate publishing course. With 1 week left to go, she received two phone calls. The first call was sobering. The second call was to let her know she better grab the next flight home. That was a long, lonely flight, without any phone or internet access for 6 hours. When she landed, she was nervous about turning her phone on. If there were good news, she would have a bunch of texts and emails. But an absence of texts and emails would mean that it was bad news, because no one would deliver bad news via texts or email. So she turned on her phone and waited. Nothing. But when she saw Alex at the airport, he told her that I was still alive, albeit in a coma. Turns out that while I wasn't dead, his phone apparently was.

Emily is a sophomore at Northwest University, studying to be a nurse. My first day or two in the hospital produced some doubts for her as she observed the ICU nurses. She began to feel as if she might not be cut out to be a nurse. But she quickly had a renewed sense of calling that not only was she going to be nurse someday, but she was "going to be a good one." Through social media, reports started coming in from all over the country, and then all over the world, of people praying for me. Emily took the lead in keeping track by placing hearts on a map. When the clouds finally lifted on day 12 of my ordeal, I saw all these heart-shaped stickers on a global map that indicated people praying for me. For me? Wow! Talk about humbling. It also turned out to be a nice geography refresher, even though she still hasn't found Guam.

Bethany is in her senior year at Puyallup High School and her second year at Pierce in their Running Start program. She's on her way to an AA degree. She loves the world of musical theater and was all set for opening weekend of *Beauty and the Beast* when my event happened. The local theater company, ManeStage, covered for her, but left her spot open to step back in when she was ready. That was awesome of them, because she was eventually able to slip back into her role, and I actually hobbled in to the final performance during closing weekend. If you were to ask Bethany what the biggest thing to happen to our family this past year was, she would look at you with a confused look as to why you would even ask, because it's obvious the retweet she got from Allie X, an indie singer, comes in at number one on the list. I have no idea who that is, but it made her year.

I love my four daughters so much. They mean the world to me. During my hospitalization, they showed a resilience, faithfulness, maturity, love, and commitment to me; to Cheryl; and to one another that impacted a lot of people. A dear friend of ours who was by our side the entire time told us that Robyn was a "rock star" for her focused demeanor throughout. Our creative writing daughter, Adria, posted some amazing updates on Facebook, and someday she'll share with me the letter to God she wrote during her flight home stating the reasons why I should live. Future nurse Emily looked over the shoulders of the ICU nurses and kept track of lines, fluids, medicines, and so on, while constantly updating the prayer map. Bethany helped out Emily with the prayer map and posted scripture verses, photos, and pictures on the walls of my hospital room. They say the man who is blessed with daughters will never have to worry about being cared for in his old age, and I got an insight into that a little sooner than I'd expected.

As for Cheryl, my wife, my BFF, and my bae, what can I say? She saved my life. How cool is that? To truly save your spouse's life is the epitome of a marital drop-the-mic moment. I'm sure that when she took that CPR class, she never imagined she would perform it someday on her husband. From now on, she gets to pick all the movies, choose the restaurants, and decide if the toilet paper roll goes over the top or down the wall. While this latest chapter in our 26-year marriage has been difficult at times, to say the least, we are currently in a great spot and excited for this new lease on life we've been given. Cheryl – I love you, I love you, I love you!

Finally, I want to say thanks to my family, friends, coworkers, and customers. Your cards, words of encouragement, emails, text messages, and Facebook comments meant more than you will ever know. I've gone back and read them, and I'm not ashamed to admit I cried like a baby. A long time ago, Jesus wept when his friend Lazarus died. Many people have nicknamed me Lazarus, including my doctors, which is awesome that they recognize that something else was going on during my recovery. That "something" was you, the hearts on the map. Just like Jesus brought Lazarus back to life, I absolutely believe I'm still here today because of your prayers. How cool is that? You played a role in saving a life, my life! So, thank you. And Merry Christmas.

I Think Lady Gaga Made My Heart Stop
By Lori Baughman-Lassen

I'm told August 19, 2010, was a great day. A day, apparently, where I drove 60 miles with my daughter and her friend to attend a Lady Gaga concert! I'm told I wasn't feeling well, complaining of neck pain. I was still not feeling great, I think, when I sat up on the edge of my bed around 5 a.m. the next morning, pausing for a bit before I went into my bathroom. I think I sat on the edge of my bathtub (because I was not feeling good?) and fell into my bathtub and, y'know, died. For some reason, my normally soundly sleeping husband heard me fall. He rushed in and couldn't find a pulse. He raced to my 15-year-old daughter's room (passing our sons' room, where my 8- and 9-year-olds were fast asleep) to tell her to call 911. He got back to me and began CPR. His only training was 16 years earlier, when I made him take a class prior to our first child being born. He did well. He kept my blood flowing until paramedics arrived 7–8 minutes later and shocked me twice. I remember nothing – from about 3 days before it happened, until I came out of the fog over 3 weeks later.

I was transported to our local hospital, which, thankfully, has a top-notch cardiac department. My sisters and mom met my husband there. Terrified, my RN oldest sister was in my room watching the ER team work flawlessly to save my life. Cold packs all around me, IVs started, monitors hooked up...What had happened? Absolutely no heart issues ever in my life. I was put on hypothermic treatment, and a hole was drilled above my forehead to monitor my brain activity. I was kept cold for a day or two, then kept in a medically induced coma for 10 days. When I was slowly brought out, no one knew how the lack of oxygen would have affected me. I was high functioning, working 8+ hours/day, raising 3 kids. I had my BA, JD, and 25 years in administration in long-term care. Would I remember that? Would I remember my family? My babies? No one knew. My sisters tell me that the past came back to me within about 24 hours. I asked where my dad was and had to be told he had died 4 years earlier. I wept, not remembering that loss. I was calm but confused. Paranoid one night that people were going to hurt me, so my sister stayed the night. My poor family went through 3 weeks of not knowing if I'd live or die and who I'd be when I did wake up.

The recovery was relatively quick. An implantable cardioverter-defibrillator was implanted a few days before I was discharged. The week after I woke up in the hospital until I was discharged is all foggy to me. Peaceful, but foggy. I don't remember feeling scared or worried. I think I was kind of in shock. I didn't understand what had happened over the past 3 weeks. I went into the hospital the morning of August 20 and returned home on my daughter's first day of high school on September 7. Using a walker for assistance for a day or two, seeing an occupational therapist and physical therapist, who saw little deficit, but I felt totally different. I didn't trust my body anymore. It had unexpectedly failed me. No warning. I have twitching almost daily; I have fallen over a dozen times (some requiring stitches) because my legs, and body, don't always respond like they used to. My speech is slower, but no one notices. I can't find words sometimes, but I compensate by quickly coming up with a new one. But, there's a new sense of lack of trust. I do, however, also feel like I can do anything if I lived through that. And, I also feel like I can take nothing for granted.

I know the ICD will prevent it from happening again, but I analyze things. I need answers – why had it happened? And, now what? Why did I survive, when so many don't? I still haven't figured that one out yet. But, I'm here. I've seen my kids have birthdays, and they're now 23, 19 and 17. Two are in college, and one is headed there this fall. I'm happy I didn't leave them. I'm happy to be alive.

Just Wanted to Take a Bath!
By Linda Hartleben-Wonder

The morning of Wednesday, February 18, 2015, began as a normal day for me and my husband, Ron. I did have a slight headache that morning, but a little coffee before my bath helped. We had the day off to take my mother-in-law to a surgical appointment, and we were getting ready for the day. However, my morning was cut short while I was in the bathtub. I do not have any memory of that day or for 4 days after and still do not understand how you can be fine one second and pulseless the next. Most of this was told to me by my husband.

My husband was blow-drying his hair in the same bathroom that I was taking a bath in and noticed that I was breathing funny and making a strong noise. He saw my color wasn't good and threw water on my face, with no response. He assumed I was having a heart attack and called 911, who coached him through CPR until first responders were able to arrive. Fortunately for me, an EMT who is a neighbor heard the call and arrived immediately, even before the ambulance. I found out later that a train was coming through

Carroll and they had to go around the train safety arms to get to me quickly. Now just the sound of a train whistle makes me pause. Our neighbor took over CPR and then tended to my husband while the ambulance crew worked to revive me. I was shocked 6 times with still showing no pulse. My veins had collapsed, so an IV was drilled into the bone of my leg. They still transported me by ambulance to the hospital in town.

When I arrived at St. Anthony's emergency department in Carroll, Dr. Kyle Ulveling, cardiologist, joined the ambulance and emergency room staff to help stabilize me, guessing I had been without oxygen for close to 16 minutes. As soon as I entered the hospital, they cooled my body to reduce brain damage, and I was prepared to be transported by *Mercy One* to Des Moines, Iowa. I was placed into a drug-induced coma and was slowly awakened the next day. I know my family was told that I might not make it – then they were told I was going to make it but probably would have a brain injury. I can credit many perfect scenarios and coming in contact with many people that day that helped me to recover "almost" completely. I don't know how anyone ever completely recovered from something like this. To top it off I didn't have any heart damage other than a left bundle branch block, but nothing else. It was all electrical – sudden cardiac arrest – Ventricular Fibrillation. I was waiting and wanting answers but never really got them. My heart quivered and stopped pumping blood for no reason; that's it. I question maybe a medication I had been on 1 month prior to my SCA might have caused it, but there was no proving that.

My road to recovery continued with Dr. Ulveling, and I started St. Anthony's cardiac rehabilitation program. I was nervous to step on a treadmill after the incident, even though I exercised a lot before. The patience, kindness, and knowledge the cardiac rehab nurses gave me were amazing. They were a big part of my recovery both mentally and physically.

The support of so many people, throughout the entire process, will not soon be forgotten. I am back to my old self with just a little different outlook on life and what's important. You never know the support system you have in place until something like this happens. It has given me peace to handle whatever may come.

Since my cardiac arrest, my husband tells me, "See you in the morning!" each night before we go to sleep. It's such a simple statement, but it is now a promise that has big meaning to us.

A big part of my personal healing has been to learn more about sudden cardiac arrest and start helping the American Heart Association. Another was to get in touch with as many people that helped me through this as I could. I have been able to do that in my hometown. I was invited to speak at the Mercy Hospital Awards Night and tell my story. I was humbled and honored to be able to get this opportunity to personally thank the Mercy Medical doctors, nurses, and staff for their help in making my story a successful one. I was also given a flight on the *Mercy One* transport helicopter and got to sit in the front seat instead of being a patient in the back! What an honor to meet the crew of *Mercy One* and to get to take a flight that I do remember!

I Experienced Sudden Cardiac Arrest While Swimming
By Carol Mathewson

On August 17, 2008, I participated in the Danskin Triathlon in Seattle and experienced sudden cardiac arrest during the swimming portion. About 20 yards from shore, I hung on to a man's kayak for a minute and then let go and sank to the bottom of the lake. Two volunteer rescue divers got me in their boat and immediately started CPR and got me to shore, where two bike medics took over. The two bike paramedics gave me two shots, intubated me, and continued CPR. Then the paramedic and firefighters arrived, shocked me two times with an AED, and got me to Harborview Hospital.

At the hospital, they put me in a medically induced coma, for 3 days, and cooled my body temperature down before bringing it back up. I had an anoxic brain injury and spent 23 days in the hospital, where I had physical therapy, occupation therapy, and speech therapy and had an implantable cardioverter-defibrillator implanted. When I returned home, I had 5 weeks of intensive PT, OT, and speech therapy at my house, followed by 6 months of PT, OT, and speech therapy, as an outpatient, before returning to work. I still have spasticity in my left hand and arm but life is great! Thanks be to God!

My Oldest Daughter, Ilissa Clark
By Tracy Clark

On February 1, 2018, my oldest daughter, 26 years old at the time, experienced her first SCA (SCD is what we recently saw on some of her paperwork as a diagnosis – sudden cardiac death, successfully resuscitated), while at work as a general manager of a popular restaurant, as she turned to go into a meeting with all the higher-ups (HR, VP, district manager, and owner). As she was going down, her face hit a table, causing her nose to break. My middle daughter was there working as well, but they wouldn't let her near her sister because she was 8 months pregnant with twins and I'm sure the scene was horrible. My middle daughter called me to let me know that her sister had passed out and the paramedics had been called. No one in the restaurant performed CPR (not even "hands only") and they didn't have an AED onsite. The lady giving orders was a trained state tested nurse aide, so I'm not sure why she didn't. Maybe all the blood from my daughter's nose scared her. When Bedford EMS arrived, my daughter had been down approximately 10 minutes without oxygen. She was taken to the nearest hospital, and a trach was placed. She was experiencing posturing and spastic movement of her limbs. They decided they weren't equipped for her situation. We followed the ambulance to the second hospital, where my middle daughter and I were given the news that her situation was grim and her chances of survival were slim (We still didn't know that she experienced an SCA at that time; the doctor didn't mention it). I felt like I had been dropped down a black hole. I made calls informing other family of the news we just received. She was taken up to ICU. Our entire family arrived, we gathered in the nurses' training room, and the floor doctor and head nurse came in to officially give us the news that she wasn't going to make it. Other family and friends braved a snowstorm that night to come out to sit and *pray* with us. They placed her in a hypothermic coma and told us whatever state she was in after 36 hours would be her state 6 months from now. I never lost faith. The third morning at shift change, the nurse came in, grabbed her light to check for pupil activity...*We had action!* She was on her way back! She slowly came to and started asking for ice in a very low whisper (they had removed the trach earlier that morning). Once she seemed alert enough the nurse began asking her if she knew where she was. She named another hospital and that she was there to have a baby and asked whether it was time to push (Her youngest was 4 at the time, but that was the last time she remembered being in a hospital). Fast-forward 23 days, lots and lots of testing. She had an implantable cardioverter-defibrillator placed the day before she left the hospital. No root cause was identified at that time, just that she had arrhythmias that most likely had sent her into arrest. She experienced her second arrest on October 7, 2018, and spent a week in the hospital. Thank God for the ICD, which shocked her three times and brought her back. Genetic testing was done. Nothing was found. After more testing it was found that she has mitral valve prolapse (MVP), and we are currently awaiting confirmation that she is a candidate for an ablation. She has returned almost 100% (she doesn't remember approximately a week before or a week or so after going down, but otherwise she's fine brain wise). Emotionally she's going through it. Hopefully she will join this group as well. And we're both in therapy. Posttraumatic stress disorder has been an issue for me. I've been living in the "What If" phase for the past year. Hopefully new ventures I've recently undertaken will help.

I've since gotten certified in CPR and AED and will be starting classes tomorrow to become an EKG technician, something I'd never thought of before this! Every October, (which is sudden cardiac arrest awareness month) we will be Bowling for Beats to bring awareness for CPR and AED training in the workplace! *I love my daughter*, and every day I count my blessings that she is still here with us. She is in "The Great 8" ❣ (Only 8% of people who experience an SCA survive!) God is great.

Our Mother
By Nathaniel Brown, Britany Thomas, & Whitney Brown

I honestly hadn't thought about how this affected me until now. As I recall the Sunday morning, I had just hung up from a short conversation with my mom. She called me, excited because she was finishing training for a 10-mile race. She was listening to the song "Happy" by Pharrell Williams on repeat and decided to call me because she was tired of hearing it. Seconds after we hung up, my phone rang again. I didn't answer because it was her number and I figured it was accidental. But it continued to ring, so I answered. It was a lady on the phone telling me my mom had just collapsed and I needed to get there. Watching my mom recover from this has been a blessing. It really has shown me the strength she has. It has also brought my little sisters and me closer together. We were very scared at the hospital that week and had to rely on each other. To be honest, I now don't like missing any of my mom's calls. It's a horrible feeling thinking that I could have never heard her voice again. That is a scary feeling that

I wouldn't wish on anyone. Although this was a tragic experience for all four of us, I now look at it as a blessing. My mom's cardiac arrest brought us closer. –Nate

My mother's SCA flipped my world upside down. During this time I had just graduated graduate school and was working in St. Louis, Missouri. It just so happened that exact weekend I was in Michigan for a wedding. I was 1 hour away when I got the call from my crying baby sister. First thought, immediate panic! One of my close friends rushed me to Hurley Medical Center, where I found my mom attached to all the proper equipment, a super swollen face, but ultimately in extremely stable condition. That's when I relaxed and was calm for the remainder of the long months of recovery. I did not return to work. I was a PRN (as-needed) worker there for the summer, and they were kind enough to release me from my contract. I went back to get my things when my mother was awake, talking, and coherent. Since then, the family has been quite protective of my mom. For one, she has posttraumatic stress disorder to the highest degree. So small things, like traveling alone, driving alone, are all concerns. Luckily my baby sister agreed to stay with my mom to help out. My brother is also very close and just a call away. But life has been a whirlwind! Overall, we are just blessed beyond measure to still have her here with us! God provides! –Britany

With my mom having SCA, it scared me and still does. You never want to see someone so close to you be in pain or near death. It affected me because now I don't like my mom being at the store alone or out and about too long for fear the same thing can happen again. I pray the device that is placed in her keeps her with us for many more years to come! –Whitney

Bibliography

Allan, C. (2013, October 2). A brush with death focused my mind. *The Guardian*. Retrieved from https://www.theguardian.com/society/2013/oct/02/brush-death-focused-mind-mortality

Baltimore Sun staff. (2019, February 28). Full transcript: Rep. Elijah Cummings' closing statements at Michael Cohen hearing. *Baltimore Sun*. Retrieved from https://www.baltimoresun.com/news/maryland/politics/bs-md-cummings-transcript-20190228-story.html

Blackwell, A. (2009, May 18). Built to last: How to keep your faith strong. Retrieved from http://www.thebridgemaker.com/how-to-keep-your-faith-strong/

Cedars-Sinai. (n.d.). *Amyloidosis.* Retrieved https://www.cedars-sinai.edu/Patients/Health-Conditions/Amyloidosis.aspx

Emerson Hospital. (n.d.). *Diagnostic testing.* Retrieved from https://www.emersonhospital.org/clinical-services/cardiology/diagnostic-testing

Holm, G. (2018). *Mitral valve prolapse (MVP)*. Retrieved from
  https://www.healthline.com/health/mitral-valve-prolapse

Hypertrophic cardiomyopathy: Optimism tinged with caution. (2011, April). *Harvard Health Letter.* Retrieved from
  https://www.health.harvard.edu/heart-health/hypertrophic-cardiomyopathy-optimism-

Stanford Health Care. (n.d.). *Alcohol septal ablation for HCM.* Retrieved from
https://stanfordhealthcare.org/medical-clinics/hypertrophic-cardiomyopathy-center/treatments.html

WJRT/TV ABC 12 *Back from illness-Crim-racer-gets 2nd chance-to cross finish line.* (2016, November). Retrieved from
  https://www.abc12.com/content/news/Back-from-illness-Crim-racer-gets-2nd-chance-to-cross-finish-line-399937091.html

APPENDIX A:

Frequently Asked Questions With Links

1. What is sudden cardiac arrest?
   https://www.sca-aware.org/sudden-cardiac-arrest-faqs#faq1

2. Is SCA the same as a heart attack?
   https://www.sca-aware.org/sudden-cardiac-arrest-faqs#faq2

3. Who is at risk for SCA? https://www.sca-aware.org/sudden-cardiac-arrest-faqs#faq3

4. What is an ejection fraction?
   https://www.sca-aware.org/sudden-cardiac-arrest-faqs#faq14

5. What causes SCA in young people?
   https://www.sca-aware.org/sudden-cardiac-arrest-faqs#faq4

6. How can SCA be prevented?
   https://www.sca-aware.org/sudden-cardiac-arrest-faqs#faq15

7. How should SCA be treated?
    https://www.sca-aware.org/sudden-cardiac-arrest-faqs#faq5

8. What is an AED? https://www.sca-aware.org/sudden-cardiac-arrest-faqs#faq16

9. How does an AED work?
    https://www.sca-aware.org/sudden-cardiac-arrest-faqs#faq7

10. Who can use an AED? https://www.sca-aware.org/sudden-cardiac-arrest-faqs#faq8

11. Can I hurt myself or others with an AED?
    https://www.sca-aware.org/sudden-cardiac-arrest-faqs#faq10

12. Are there special considerations when placing electrodes on a female victim?
    https://www.sca-aware.org/sudden-cardiac-arrest-faqs#faq12

13. What if the victim has a medication patch, such as nitroglycerin? https://www.sca-aware.org/sudden-cardiac-arrest-faqs#faq13

14. What if the victim has an implantable pacemaker or defibrillator? https://www.sca-aware.org/sudden-cardiac-arrest-faqs#faq17

15. Do AEDs always help SCA victims? https://www.sca-aware.org/sudden-cardiac-arrest-faqs#faq18

16. Do I have to have a prescription to acquire an AED? https://www.sca-aware.org/sudden-cardiac-arrest-faqs#faq22

17. Do AEDs replace the use of CPR? https://www.sca-aware.org/sudden-cardiac-arrest-faqs#faq21

18. After resuscitation, will the victim be able to resume a normal life? https://www.sca-aware.org/sudden-cardiac-arrest-faqs#faq23

19. Can AEDs be used to treat children?
https://www.sca-aware.org/sudden-cardiac-arrest-faqs#faq24

20. Can you live a normal life after cardiac arrest?
https://www.npr.org/sections/health-shots/2013/03/14/174291275/cardiac-arrest-survivors-have-better-outlook-than-doctors-think

21. What happens to the brain after cardiac arrest?   https://journalofethics.ama-assn.org/article/prognosis-and-therapy-after-cardiac-arrest-induced-coma/2009?08

22. What happens during therapeutic hypothermia after cardiac arrest?
https://www.hopkinsmedicine.org/healthlibrary/test_procedures/cardiovascular/therapeutic_hypothermia_after_cardiac_arrest_135,393

23. What is the most common cause of sudden cardiac arrest?
https://www.mayoclinic.org/diseases-conditions/sudden-cardiac-arrest/symptoms-causes/syc-20350634

24. What is the difference between cardiac
    arrests and heart attacks?
     https://www.heart.org/en/health-
    topics/heart-attack/about-heart-
    attacks/heart-attack-or-sudden-cardiac-
    arrest-how-are-they-different

25. Is sudden cardiac death hereditary?
    https://blog.oup.com/2013/04/sudden-
    cardiac-death-heart-family/

26. Can sudden cardiac death be prevented?
    https://www.medicinenet.com/sudden_
    cardiac_death/article.htm

27. How long does it take to die from cardiac
    arrest?
    https://www.verywellhealth.com/brain-
    activity-after-cardiac-arrest-1298429

28. Can palpitations cause cardiac arrest?
    https://universityhealthnews.com/daily
    /heart-health/cardiac-arrest-symptoms/

APPENDIX B:

SCA Articles & Case Studies

Sudden cardiac arrest - Test your heart health IQ
https://www.emedicinehealth.com/sudden_cardiac_arrest_death_quiz_iq/faq.htm

The impact of cardiac arrest on the long-term wellbeing and caregiver burden of family caregivers: A prospective cohort study
https://www.ncbi.nlm.nih.gov/pubmed/28068794

Care for the adult family members of victims of unexpected cardiac death
https://onlinelibrary.wiley.com/doi/pdf/10.1197/j.aem.2006.06.029

Teaching CPR to families of heart patients before they leave the hospital
https://www.pcori.org/research-results/2015/teaching-cpr-families-heart-patients-they-leave-hospital

When heart disease turns traumatic – PTSD
https://www.health.harvard.edu/newsletter_article/When_heart_disease_turns_traumatic

Hands-only CPR
https://cpr.heart.org/AHAECC/CPRAndECC/Programs/HandsOnlyCPR/UCM_473196_Hands-Only-CPR.jsp

Surviving a sudden cardiac arrest...Now what?
http://www.suddencardiacarrest.org/aws/SCAA/asset_manager/get_file/32772?ver=859

APPENDIX C:

Support Groups & Resources

Sudden Cardiac Arrest Foundation
https://www.sca-aware.org/

Sudden Cardiac Arrest Association
http://www.suddencardiacarrest.org/aws/SCAA/pt/sp/home_page

Arrhythmia Alliance
http://www.heartrhythmalliance.org/aa/us/sudden-cardiac-arrest

Sudden Cardiac Arrest Association | Education Materials
http://www.suddencardiacarrest.org/aws/SCAA/pt/sp/edmaterials

Heart Health Project
http://www.heartrescueproject.com/community-sca-response-planning-guide/survivor-support/patient-support-reintegration/support-groups/

Sudden Cardiac Arrest Survivors Support Group on Facebook. [You need a Facebook account in order to access this group].
https://www.facebook.com/

S.C.A. Survivors Support Group on Facebook. [You need a Facebook account in order to access this group]. https://www.facebook.com/

APPENDIX D:

Songs to Do CPR To

According to The New York-Presbyterian Hospital Ronald O. Perelman Heart Institute to be effective, perform hands-only CPR at a pace of 100 or 120 beats per minute (BPM). How will you know if you are performing at a rate of 100/120 BPM? The New York-Presbyterian Hospital Ronald O. Perelman Heart Institute compiled the following list of 100/120 BPM songs. Find a song that you like, memorize it, and when that time ever comes for you to perform CPR, think of the song and silently sing it to yourself as you apply pressure to the chest of a victim. Learn more at https://www.nyp.org/cpr/.

1. Just Dance by Lady Gaga, Colby O'Donis * The Fame Monster (Deluxe)
2. Something Just Like This by The Chainsmokers, Coldplay * Something Just Like This
3. Rumour Has It by Adele * 21
4. Sorry by Justin Bieber * Purpose (Deluxe)
5. Hang With Me by Robyn * Body Talk

6. Okay by Holy Ghost! * Dynamics
7. Closer by POWERS * Closer
8. Say You'll Be There by Spice Girls * Spice
9. I Will Survive – Remastered by Gloria Gaynor
    * Gloria Gaynor (Remastered)
10. Rock Your Body by Justin Timberlake *
    Justified
11. Stayin' Alive by Bee Gees * Staying Alive
    (Original motion picture soundtrack)
12. Cecilia by Simon & Garfunkel * Greatest Hits
13. Hard to Handle by The Black Crowes *
    Greatest Hits 1990?1999: A Tribute to a Work
    in Progress
14. Sweet Home Alabama by Lynyrd Skynyrd *
    Second Helping
15. MMMBop – Single Version by Hanson * The
    Best of Hanson: 20th Century Masters: The
    Millennium Collection
16. Gives You Hell by The All-American Rejects *
    When the World Comes Down
17. Heartbreaker by Mariah Carey, Jay Z *
    Rainbow
18. Who's That Girl by Madonna * Celebration
    (double disc version)
19. Fast Car by Tracy Chapman * Tracy Chapman
20. Fly by Sugar Ray * Rhino Hi-Five: Sugar Ray

21. Rock This Town – Single Edit/24 Bit Mastering/Digital Remaster/1999 by Stray Cats * The Brian Setzer Collection 1981?1988 (Remastered)

22. Hips Don't Lie by Shakira, Wyclef Jean * Oral Fixation, Vol. 2 (Expanded edition)

23. You Can't Hurry Love – 2016 Remastered by Phil Collins * Hello, I Must Be Going! (Deluxe edition)

24. Notorious B.I.G. (feat. Lil' Kim & Puff Daddy) by The Notorious B.I.G., Lil' Kim, and Diddy * Born Again (Explicit)

25. Work It by Missy Elliott * Under Construction (Explicit)

26. What's Going On by Marvin Gaye * The Complete Collection

27. Suddenly I See by KT Tunstall * Eye to the Telescope

28. Five to One by The Doors * Waiting for the Sun

29. Crazy by Gnaris Barkley * St. Elsewhere

30. Spirit in the Sky by Norman Greenbaum * Music from the Motion Picture Michael

31. Girls Just Want to Have Fun by Cyndi Lauper * Twelve Deadly Cyns...And Then Some

32. The Book of Love by The Monotones * Who Wrote the Book of Love?(Digital version)

33. (Sittin'On) The Dock of the Bay by Otis Redding * Atlantic 60th: Soul, Sweat and Strut

34. Ain't No Mountain High Enough (feat. Marvin Gaye and Diana Ross) by Kris King * The Beat Arsenal Vol. 1

35. This Ain't a Scene, It's an Arms Race by Fall Out Boy * Believers Never Die – Greatest Hits

36. Body Movin' by Beastie Boys, Fatboy Slim * Hello Nasty (Deluxe version/remastered 2009) (Explicit)

37. Walk Like an Egyptian by The Bangles * The Essential Bangles

38. Dancing Queen by ABBA * ABBA Gold

39. Heart and Soul by T'Pau * 80's Super Hits

40. Another Brick in the Wall, Pt. 2 by Pink Floyd * The Wall

41. Quit Playing Games (With My Heart) by Backstreet Boys * Backstreet Boys

42. Man in the Mirror – Remastered version by Michael Jackson * Michael Jackson's This Is It

43. Hey, Soul Sister by Train * Save Me, San Francisco (Golden Gate edition)

44. Float On by Modest Mouse * Good News for People Who Love Bad News

45. Crazy in Love by Beyoncé, JAY Z * Dangerously in Love

46. One Week by Barenaked Ladies * Stunt (20th anniversary edition)
47. History of Rap (feat. Justin Timberlake) by Jimmy Fallon and Justin Timberlake * Blow Your Pants Off

APPENDIX E:

How do you keep your faith strong?
By Alex Blackwell

1. Allow yourself to grieve for what you have lost.
2. Be patient with the uncertainty.
3. Watch how you rebound and fill in the gaps.
4. Faith is resistible; learn not to resist, but to receive more.
5. Get involved.
6. Focus on the positive.
7. Have deep water faith in the shallow end.

Photos & Articles of my Journey

Hurley Medical Center -
August 14-17, 2016 ~ The Day I Forgot

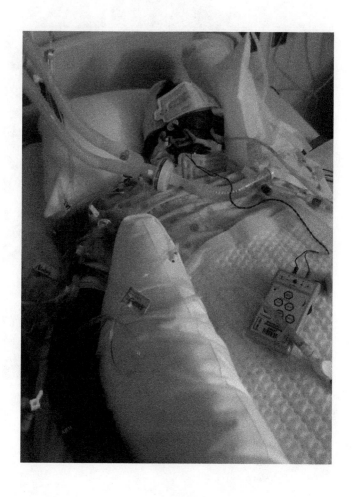

Hurley Medical Center -
August 14-17, 2016 ~ The Day I Forgot

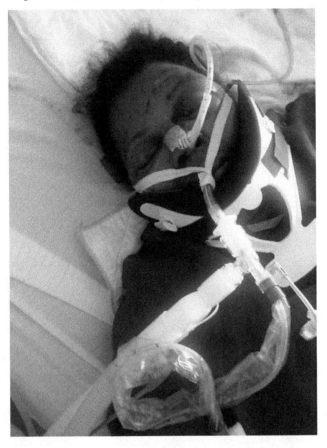

U of M Survival Flight - August 17, 2016, I was airlifted to University of Michigan Hospital in Ann Arbor, Michigan for specialized treatment of my orbital bone fracture and SCA.

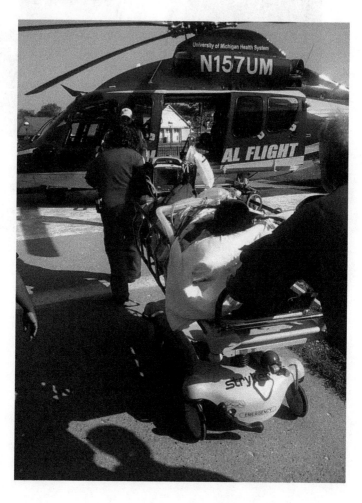

Gina Russell, RN, was one of my survival flight nurses to U of M Hospital in Ann Arbor!

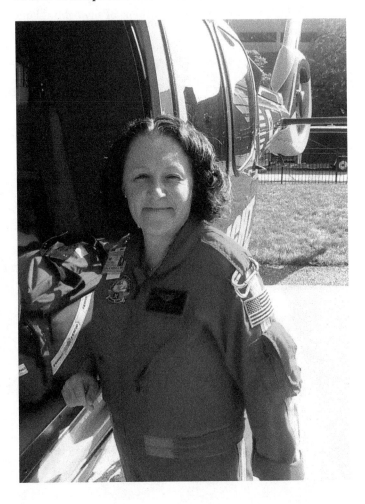

My ICU nurse had me up each day, sitting in my chair and walking the hallways.

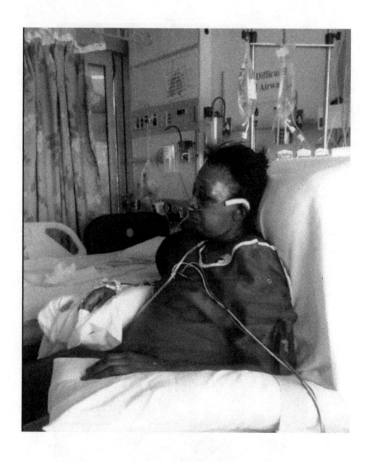

August 26, 2016: Crim Festival of Races Day, my Pastor, Jeffery Hawkins, Sr., walked the 10-mile route in tribute to me.

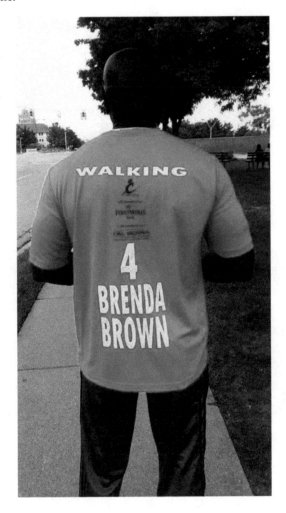

August 26, 2016: Crim Festival of Races Day, my team leader, Debra Collins walked the 10-mile route in tribute to me.

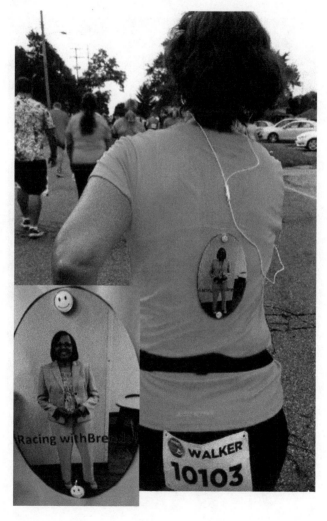

On August 26, 2016: My version of race day with my children in the hospital as I walked the hospital hallways.

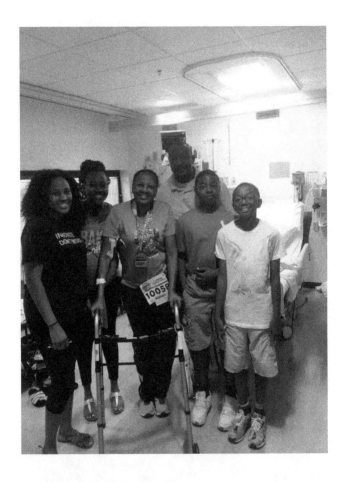

My children "Expressions of Joy" during my recovery!

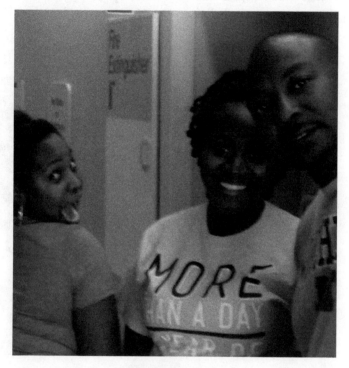

Blessed By Three

The three of you will never know how much my love has grown for you behind this traumatic event that impacted our lives. You all are my life and my joy.

I am blessed to have the three of you in my life.

May God continue to bless us all!

November 3, 2016 – The Crim Foundation gave me an opportunity to finish the Crim Road Race...two months after I had collapsed. I had a whole group of people supporting me, including my son (Nate), my daughter (Whitney) , my brother (Lee),my uncle (Roosevelt Brown) my pastor (Jeffey Hawkins, Sr.), many friends, and Crim Race Director, Andrew Younger.

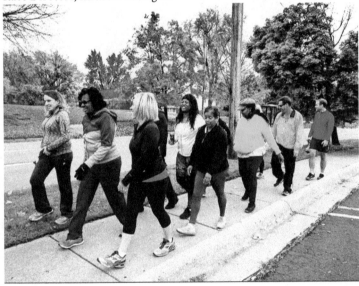

November 3, 2016 – My fellow "Crimmers" who walked with me as I finished what I had started. **Pictured L to R:** Lynn Reynolds, Jennifer Follett, Brenda Brown, Debra Collins, Carol Raznic, John Collins and Dee-Dee Hurley.

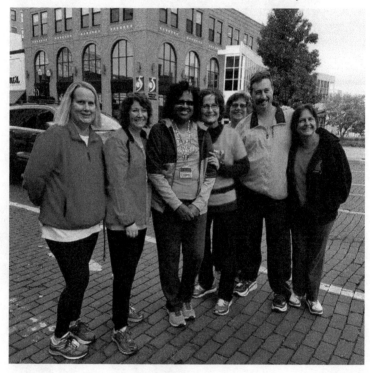

Andrew Younger, Crim Foundation, presenting me with my medal. **Below:** I was thanking Ashley & Renee Race again for saving my life.

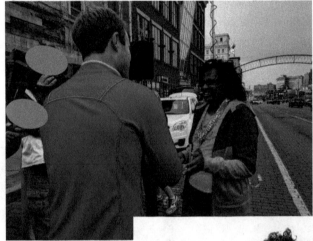

November 3, 2016 – My team leader and friend, Debra Collins and I posing for a quick picture before heading to finish the race I had started.

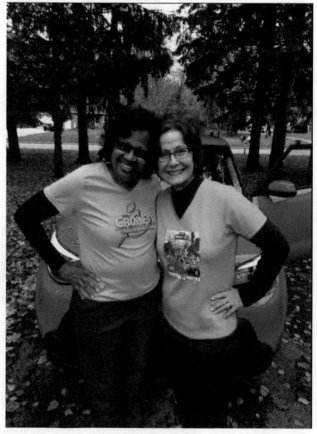

Dee-Dee and I waiting to finish to race I had started.
Below: John wishing me luck as I was about to embark on
my 1.2 mile trek.

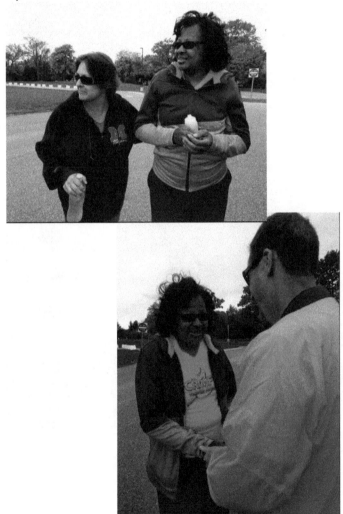

FlintSide ALEXANDRIA BROWN | WEDNESDAY, JANUARY 30, 2019 | *Flintside*

After surviving death, this Flint woman raises awareness of hidden, often deadly, heart condition

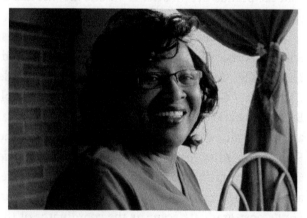

Brenda Brown is writing a book titled, "The Day I Forgot But Will Always Remember."

Flint, Michigan — Brenda Brown, 61, is not a woman of confrontation. Her voice is soft and never rises above a certain volume. She has a way of speaking with a continuous smile that immediately puts a person at ease. Though she is not one for confrontation, make no mistake about it: She is a fighter.

You see, Brenda Brown died two years ago.

But, she fought her way back — surviving Sudden Cardiac Arrest in August 2016 and becoming a strong voice to educate others about the medical condition.

"There was a Brenda Brown before this," she says. "But the Brenda Brown after is the one that life had to change."

The Brenda before is a twin and one of 11 siblings. She was born in Flint and moved to Otisville as a child. There, she and her siblings attended LakeVille Community Schools. After graduating high school, Brown embarked on an encompassing professional and academic career that would bring her back to the Flint area. After earning degrees from Hillsdale College, Central Michigan University, Baker College, and Capella University, Brown immersed herself in Flint's post-graduate scene as the coordinator of the Academic Resource Center at Baker College.

She was a mother of three and loved her job. She woke up each morning, went to work, and never much thought about what could happen to her life or death. "I didn't give any thought about if something was going to happen. It was just a guarantee," said Brown. "I never put a lot of thought into: Is tomorrow promised to me?"

On Aug. 14, 2016, Brenda's world changed.

She had been training to walk in the Crim 10-mile race. There was just two more weeks until the big race. She joined the swarms of people that celebrate the annual painting of the blue line that marks the 10-mile route by walking or running the freshly painted course.

She had previously dodged heart failure in 2007, but she underwent surgery, recovered, and was healthy — fit to walk and ready to celebrate her health.

She, like many Crim athletes, dreaded as each step took her closer and closer to the Bradley Hills — a series of steep inclines on Bradley Avenue at about the 5-mile mark. Brown knew her hard work was paying off.

She walked the hills with no trouble and excitedly called her son to celebrate. The hard part was over. The biggest obstacles were behind her and she knew she still had enough energy to walk the rest of the distance.

Brown didn't recognize that by mile 7 in the Woodcroft neighborhood, she was beginning to act out of character. Benita Seale, 56, saw Brown begin to stumble after the 8 mile mark.

"That's when I noticed her, when we were on Miller Road going toward the School of the Deaf … I noticed that there was this lady (that seemed to be staggering) somewhat," said Seales. "All of the sudden, she falls."

She was just shy of the 9-mile mark of her walk. Brown doesn't remember anything about Aug. 14, 2016. She's been able to piece together the details from family, friends, and witnesses like Seale.

She knows now that she collapsed after experiencing a spontaneous heart condition called Sudden Cardiac Arrest, also called SCA. It caused her heart to stop. Completely. In an instant. She collapsed to the ground, motionless. She lost consciousness before she hit the ground and did nothing to brace for impact, smashing her face against the pavement.

Brown explains now, to anyone and everyone who will listen, that SCA is different from a heart attack. It is more an electrical problem than a plumbing problem, she says. And, more immediate. The neurons in the mind misfire and tell the heart to stop beating instantly. The causes are unknown.

"(Doctors) did not expect for me to survive, which it still freaks me out sometimes," Brown says.

Amidst frantic assistance and chest compressions by fellow racers, an ambulance was called and Brown was taken to Hurley Medical Center. Family was called and the waiting game began. Then the healing and recovery began.

She had a defibrillator implanted so that if her heart ever stops again it can be automatically given an electric shock to restart it. And, less than three months later, she returned to the Crim course and she walked the remainder of that 10-mile trek.

Life had forever changed for Brown.

"I seriously don't have bad days," says Brown. "Bad stuff can happen, but my attitude, my perception on everything, is completely different. ...I was granted a second opportunity at life. I'm not going to let little things — well, things period — get in the way of this life at this point."

Because of her condition, Brown was advised by her doctor to go on disability leave in June 2018. Now, Brown is dedicating even more time to educating people about SCA — including writing a book about her experience — and living her life, every day, knowing she could have a recurrence.

Even with a defibrillator, there remains real risk — primarily because the only way to test if the defibrillator really works is by having another cardiac arrest.

"There's a whole wide community of folks out there. ... It's supportive. It's helpful, but it's also," Brown hesitates, "It's a little scary because you hear folks say 'I've had two' and then one says 'I've had eight,'" she says. "It's mind-boggling in a way because it's like, 'Oh my goodness you've had that many?' You know, I'm thinking one and that's it for me. I don't expect to have any more."

Still, Brown always takes certain precautions. She keeps her iPhone location on at all times and makes sure the moments she is alone are far and few in between. She now shares her home on Flint's southside with her daughter and granddaughter. There she busies herself by preparing lessons for Sunday school classes at Prince of Peace Baptist Church and spends four hours a day devoted to her book.

Aptly titled, "The Day I Forgot But Will Always Remember," the book is about healing, creating a better understanding of SCA, and life for its survivors.

"It is also my reminder that my near-death experience is not the end of life but a new beginning," she says.

Article Link:

http://www.flintside.com/features/brendabrown.aspx

First Re-Birth Dinner with Rescuers & Family
November 5, 2016

My children & grandchildren celebrated my re-birth. *Back Row L to R:* Nate, Jr., Whitney, Nehemiah & Kayla. *Front Row L to R:* Nate, Sr., Nicole (7 weeks old); Brenda & Britany

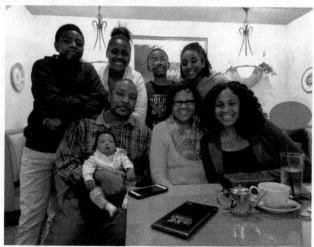

Below: My walking partner, Dee-Dee Hurley, and team leader, Debra Collins. Both ladies were by my bedside from day one. Unbeknown to me, they made numerous trips to Hurley Medical Center and UofM Hospital to sit with me.

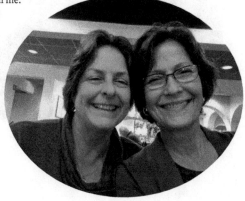

First Re-Birth Dinner with Rescuers & Family

From L to R: Dee-Dee Hurley, John Collins, Ashley Knific, Brenda Brown, Renee McMann, Benita Seale, Randy Seale, April Hawkins, and Pastor Jeffery Hawkins. Sr.

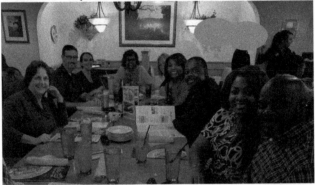

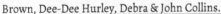

Below: Third Re-Birth Dinner. **L to R:** Britany Thomas, Brenda Brown, Dee-Dee Hurley, Debra & John Collins.

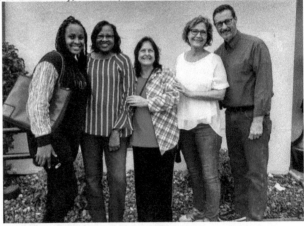

First Dinner with Rescuers & Family
November 5, 2016

Left: John Collins, Ashley Knific, Brenda Brown & Rene McMann. I will be forever grateful to these angels for not giving up on me. ***Below left:*** My Pastor & his wife, Pastor Jeffery & Sis. April Hawkins, Sr. His spiritual direction helped deepened my relationship with God during my recovery.

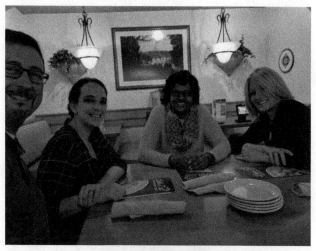

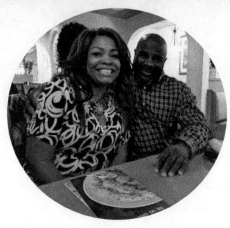

Hurley Medical Center
Cardiac Rehabilitation - 2018

As I continued my road to recovery, there were days when I felt like giving up. But my cardiac rehabilitation nurse, Nicole Richey, and Exercise Physiologist, Jouroin Szczepaniak, kept me and others patients motivated with their kind words and loving spirit. This particular Thought of the Week *"IF IT DOESN'T CHALLENGE YOU, IT WON'T CHANGE YOU"* motivated me to continue on with my treatment plan!

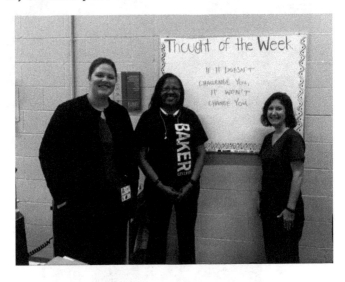

Long story short:

"Cardiac Rehab helps heart patients feel better."

ABOUT THE AUTHOR

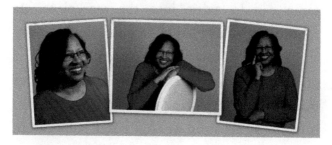

Brenda Brown is a mother of three and grandmother of five. She is a twin and one of 11 living siblings. Her willingness to serve and to help people is captured even in her career goal to "help students to succeed and be prepared for the economic and social opportunities that will empower them as individuals." She practices what she preaches. Her parents instilled in Brenda and her siblings the importance of education. Though she encountered many hurdles – including racial, social, and economic – she persevered, earning an associate, bachelor's, master's, and then doctoral degree. She held the same high expectations for her children, whom she inspired to achieve higher education degrees. Brenda carries that same can-do spirit into the workplace. As coordinator of Academic Resource Center, daily she guides and encourages students, regardless of their circumstances, to grow and learn. Her mantra is a Nelson Mandela quote: "An education is the most powerful weapon which you can use to change the world."

Beyond home and work, she believes that giving back is vital to promoting community – and she does! Her past volunteer efforts include Big Brothers Big Sisters of Greater Flint (BB/BS), the Beecher Scholarship Incentive Program, the Genesee County Reaching Across the Nation Consortium, Department of Human Services Michigan Youth Opportunity Initiatives, the Dr. Martin Luther King Jr. Tribute Dinner Planning Committee, the Gateway Cultivating Our Community garden project, and the United Way. Perhaps most notable, for over 30 years, Brenda has served as a mentor for BB/BS. She also mentored for Living Independently Networking Knowledge (L.I.N.K.), volunteered as the coordinator for her church's weekly A Taste of Tutoring program, and served as the Amachi liaison between BB/BS and her church. She has been a past mentor for West Bendle and Garfield Elementary Schools' Help One Student To Succeed (HOSTS) programs (6 years), an advisor to the Baker College Tutoring Association's tutoring programs for Flint Community Schools and Bendle Public Schools (15 years), and a former co-chair of Flint Area Citizens to End Racism Youth Action Team and Steering Committee (5 years). She has served as facilitator of the Great Lakes District Youth Leadership (1 year) and board member of Flint Leadership Development in Interethnic Relations (2 years). She also served as a member of the Flint Area Public Affairs Forum (1 year).

In all her community service Brenda brings courage, commitment, compassion, and understanding that have continued to grow from her early childhood experiences as being part of the only minority family in a small, rural community. Befriended by one White, female classmate, following high school graduation,

Brenda was determined to similarly become a champion for social justice. Her faith serves as a strong foundation. She is an active member of Prince of Peace Missionary Baptist Church, where she is a Sunday school teacher and serves in multiple ministries.

Brenda lives, works, and volunteers – demonstrating the essence of Luke 12:48 (KJV), "For unto whomsoever much is given, of him shall be much required: and to whom men have committed much, of him they will ask the more."

NOTES:

_____

_____

_____

_____

_____

_____

_____

_____

_____

_____

_____

_____

_____

_____

_____

_____

_____

_____

_____

_____

_____

_____

NOTES:

_____

_____

_____

_____

_____

_____

_____

_____

_____

_____

_____

_____

_____

_____

_____

_____

_____

_____

_____

_____

If you have questions for the author, please
contact her at bbrown9836@gmail.com

CPSIA information can be obtained
at www.ICGtesting.com
Printed in the USA
FFHW010721111019
55499274-61291FF